AYURVEDA FOR BEGINNERS- PITTA

The Only Guide You Need To Balance Your Pitta Dosha For Vitality, Joy, And Overall Well-being!!

Rohit Sahu

CONTENTS

AUTHOR NOTE

Dear Reader,

As you delve into the pages of this book, you'll notice that the images and elements are presented in black and white. This decision was made with thoughtful consideration, aimed at balancing quality, accessibility, and affordability.

Color printing, while visually appealing, comes at a significant cost, which would be reflected in a higher selling price. To keep this book within reach of as many readers as possible, I chose an economical black and white format.

However, I also recognize the added value that color brings to your reading experience, especially when it comes to appreciating delicious recipies. To ensure you don't miss out, I've provided a QR code that grants complimentary access to a digital version of the book, where these images come to life in full color.

I hope this addition enhances your experience and invites you into the world of Pitta Balancing, both on the page and beyond.

With the deepest gratitude,

Rohit Sahu

INTRODUCTION

Ayurveda, which derives from ancient Vedic scriptures, is a 5,000-year-old medical ideology and philosophy based on the idea that we are all made up of different types of energy.

There are 3 doshas in Ayurveda that describe the dominant state of mind/body—Vata, Pitta, and Kapha. While all three are present in everyone, Ayurveda suggests that we each have a dominant dosha that is unwavering from birth, and ideally an equal (though often fluctuating) balance between the other two. If doshas are balanced, we are healthy; when they are unbalanced, we develop a disorder commonly expressed by skin problems, impaired nutrition, insomnia, irritability, and anxiety.

Vata, Pitta, and Kapha are all important to our biology in some way, so no one is greater than, or superior to, any other. Each has a very specific set of basic functions to perform in the body.

Although all three doshas are present everywhere in the body, the ancient Vedic texts describe a "Home Location" for each of the doshas. "Vata is mainly found below the navel, Pitta mainly between navel and heart, and Kapha above the heart."

That said, when the doshas are out of control, our well-being can be damaged. However, before we get into the particulars of each of the three doshas, it is helpful to understand their basic nature and their wider function in the natural world.

Throughout Ayurveda, the most basic building blocks in the material world are the 5 elements—Space, Air, Fire, Water, and Earth.

Vata is characterized by the mobile nature of Air (Wind) energy.

Pitta embodies the transformative nature of Fire energy. And Kapha reflects the binding nature of Water energy.

Each of the doshas has its own special strengths and weaknesses, and with a little awareness, you can do a lot to remain healthy and balanced. You can use this 'Ayurveda For Beginners' series to adjust your lifestyles and routines in a way that supports your constitution. It consists of three parts, one for each. This is Pitta; the other two are also available.

What's the Meaning of Pitta?

To Ayurveda, Pitta is one of the three doshas—energetic forces of nature that make up the universe and everything within it, including us! Pitta is associated with the components of fire and water, but the former is more prominent. Together, they are the important power that controls the transformational processes of the body and metabolism; even the hormones of the body are believed to be regulated by Pitta.

Pitta is the hottest, oiliest, and sharpest of the three doshas. When you feel overheated in any way, there may be an abundance of the Pitta Dosha inside your body.

Pitta describes both the biological characteristics of the individual and the character of the person. The main characteristics of Pitta Dosha are hot, sharp, intense, light, bitter, and spreading. People with Pitta dominance usually have fiery bodies and minds. They are medium in size, both in height and in weight. They have good digestion and a very strong appetite and thirst.

Individuals with Pitta dominance are enthusiastic, positive, ambitious but also somewhat aggressive. They are willing to focus on the task and devote everything to its realization, which makes them leaders—they manage to organize the action of Vata and Kapha type.

According to Ayurveda, Pittas are willing, strong, dominant, creative, driven, and definitive. If Pitta is out of control, they can become irritable, furious, judgmental, hostile, and even violent. They may have an acidic stomach, oversensitive skin, extreme body pain, or heartburn.

The term 'Pitta' comes from Sanskrit, meaning 'Warmth' or 'Transformation.' When a person is born, Pitta is in harmony with the other two energies, Vata and Kapha. Each of them handles a certain portion of the other functions of the body. The Pitta governs all the different forms of digestion and transformation that manifest in our mind and body (It controls digestion and metabolism so that the fire can flare first in the small intestine and the stomach—Pitta's main body seats—with excess digestive acid and bile). The motions—the bloodstream, the breathing, the blinking, the nerve impulses, etc., and even the movements of the essential energies themselves—depend on Vata. Liquid monitoring is carried out via Kapha.

Transformation is the primary function of Pitta. As previously said, it governs all the different forms of digestion and transformation that manifest in our mind and body—from digesting sensory impressions and emotional reactions to transforming Chyle (lymph and fatty matter from partially digested food) into protoplasmic substances such as sperm and ova, and how we discriminate between right and wrong.

It is closely linked to Agni (Digestive Fire). The properties are pungent, hot, penetrating, greasy, oily, sticky, liquid, spreading, and sour. The primary locus of Pitta is the small intestine where most chemical degradation happens, but it also exists in the eyes, blood, sweat glands, stomach, and lymph.

Made up of Agni (Fire) and Jala (Water), Pitta seems to be a contradiction in words, but its two constituents are actually complementary. The liquid nature of Pitta protects the tissues from the destructive aspects of fire and enables Pitta's metabolic properties to flow through the body in fluids such as bile, digestive enzymes, and hormones.

In addition to playing an important role in the digestive and endocrine processes, Pitta influences body temperature, visual perception, appetite, thirst, and the quality of the skin.

Mentally and physically, Pitta encourages sound judgment, integrity, commitment, and happiness when in harmony. If it is out of control, it creates restlessness, rage and irritability, frustration, envy, dissatisfaction, or intense negativity. Thus, Pitta controls all metabolic processes in the body as well as the temperature of the body and our hormonal balance. Hunger, thirst, and even wisdom are connected to Pitta.

If Pitta is in balance, there are no health problems. But if Pitta is out of balance, diseases occur because the function of several organs and the types of processes is disturbed. Normally this contributes to the imbalance in the other two doshas, so a complex of diseases occurs.

To balance Pitta, it is advised to eat foods that neutralize Pitta's warm qualities. Out of balance, Pitta should resist spicy foods and heating vegetables such as garlic, onions, or chilli peppers. It is also advised to perform yoga asanas to keep Pitta in check.

Pitta has the most in common with summer. Imagine a steaming pot of hot, sour, and spicy soup—that's the nature of the Pitta. Made up of the primary elements Fire (mainly) and Water (secondary), Pitta has hot, oily, sharp, light, sour, fluid, and pungent attributes—many of the same sensory qualities that summer surrounds us.

Also, it's a fundamental principle of Ayurveda that 'Like Increases Like.' So, when summer heats up, we are vulnerable to the buildup of extra Pitta. If we already have a Pitta Prakriti (nature), we are at an even higher risk of getting out of balance.

Signs of Pitta deficiency include diarrhea, burning feelings, skin irritation, odorous sweating, fever, swelling, and hypercritical or extreme mental outlook. Excess Pitta can cause the body, mind, and emotions to feel overheated. This kind of imbalance can happen to anyone, irrespective of their Ayurvedic nature or body type.

In this book, we'll dive deeper into what Pitta means, what throws Pitta out of balance, and how to identify the Pitta Dosha in your environment, in yourself, and in others.

With this book, I'm going to share with you everything you need to know to balance your Pitta Dosha and use it for your overall vitality, joy, and well-being.

The book includes Pitta-stabilizing lifestyle tips, guidance on different Pitta-dosha diets, including what Pitta foods to skip and what to eat.

It also includes the characteristics/qualities, Pitta Dosha disorders and ways to deal with it, tastes that pacify Pitta, how to eat, and some delicious recipes. I'm even going to talk about the best yogic practices for Pitta Dosha, including pranayamas and types of asanas that Pitta Dosha should absolutely not skip.

Such tips are not intended as a strict set of rules, but rather as a practical checklist for creating a sense of order that can be easily implemented in your Pitta lifestyle.

The simplest way to balance the Pitta Dosha is by 'Following a Routine.' Whether you have a Pitta body type or you're having Pitta deficiency, a daily routine that works on counteracting Pitta's natural tendency for excessive heat and acidity can be a huge help. I'm going to walk you through how you can start tiny by sticking to a routine to work out, go to bed, and eat every meal each day.

Just follow the book along, and you'll reveal the easiest step-by-step routine to balance your Pitta Dosha by the end of it!

WHAT IS PITTA DOSHA?

itta reflects the body's heat, fire, and strength. Biologically, this is a mixture of energy and liquid. Energy functions as an active principle and liquid play a role as a medium. All biochemical functions in the body are due to the elements of Pitta. Pitta splits the Kapha molecules (complex substances) into simpler ones and then releases the energy. Pitta word is derived from 'Tapa,' which means heat, energy, or fire.

The proper volume of Pitta controls body temperature, digestion, and metabolism. But when Pitta rates rise (Excess Pitta) it may contribute to severe health problems. It's named the Pitta Dosha.

Symptoms of Pitta Dosha

Physical:

• Heightened hunger and/or thirst

• Urinary tract irritation

• Early hair loss or grey hair, greasy hair, excessive body hair growth

• Hormonal deficiency

• Giddiness and headaches/migraines

• Hot bursts and demand for things that have a cooling impact on the body

- Foul breath/body odor
- Bloated swelling, acne, cold sore throat
- Sickness when skipping meals
- Nausea
- Tenderness in breasts/testicles
- Discoloration of the skin
- Burning feelings in the body
- Sensitivity to the sun and heat
- Skin infection, e.g. swelling, acne, eczema, and dermatitis
- Digestive diseases—Acidity e.g. acid reflux, heartburn, diarrhea
- Allergies, piles, hemorrhoids, polyps
- Lack of vision, eye disorders, burning pain of the eyes
- Severe swelling of the body or joints
- Acid reflux, gastric or peptic ulcers, heartburn
- Loose stools

Behavioral:
- Impatience
- Irritation
- Excessive ego
- An intense sensation of heat in the body
- Agitation, rage, irritability
- Judgment, impatience, disapproval, intolerance

- Extreme perfectionist tendencies

- Overly targeted/result-oriented

- Dissatisfaction

- Envy

- Judgmental

- Sense of uncertainty

- Perfectionist tendencies

- Pitta-type depression, anxiety, disruptive, aggressive behavior, self-harm

- Panic attack, fainting

- Rage, envy, irritability

- High aspirations, perfectionism, judgment, criticism, obsessions

Effects in Various Parts of Body

In the Mind

Changes in the mental state—such as irritability, rage, impatience, judgment, disapproval, and envy—are all related to Pitta's imbalance. Excess Pitta in the mind may also induce an inclination towards perfectionism, or a general sense of disappointment or discontent. When Pitta is left to grow uncontrolled, it can contribute to extreme indignation, frustration, aggression, excessive envy, obsessive-compulsive behavior, and even depression.

AYURVEDA FOR BEGINNERS- PITTA

In the Blood, Skin, and Sweat

Excess Pitta can cause the skin to appear red or yellowish and warm to the touch. You can also have hives, fever, asthma, eczema, psoriasis, or dermatitis.

Excessive heat in the blood may trigger nausea, hot flashes, burning or scratching symptoms, bleeding impulses, hematomas, and hemorrhoids. It may cause people to burn or bruise quickly and raise their vulnerability towards the sun. The tongue may look bruised or swollen and there may be bleeding gums, canker sores, or ulcers in the mouth.

Excessive sweating, acid perspiration, and strong fleshy-smelling body odor are also typical manifestations of imbalance. Signs with more extreme diseases in these regions include obvious capillary networks, significant bleeding problems, hemorrhage, jaundice, hepatitis, abscess, gangrene, melanoma, lupus, gout, mononucleosis, blood clots, strokes, and myeloid leukemia.

In the Digestive Tract

Early symptoms of Pitta deficiency in the digestive system include extreme appetite, intense fatigue, and a feeling of insatiability. When Pitta builds up, it may induce nausea, vomiting, hiccups, acid reflux, heartburn, loose stools, diarrhea, low blood sugar, and allergy to spicy and/or fried foods.

The tongue can have a yellowish layer, a salty odor, or a foul, fetid-smelling breath. The waste can be greenish or yellowish, a sour scent, which can induce a burning feeling after expulsion.

Imbalanced Pitta in the digestive tract may induce extreme acid indigestion or heartburn, fatty diarrhea, stool bleeding,

9

stomach or esophagus swelling, appendicitis, and peptic ulcers.

In Other Parts of the Body

Burning red or bloodshot eyes, excessive sensitivity to light, and yellowish tincture in white eyes are also symptoms of excess Pitta. Some more symptoms are tendonitis, bursitis, muscle weakness, persistently elevated blood pressure, occasional headaches, and hair loss.

Aggravated Pitta can also induce dizziness, nausea, herpes flare-ups, shingles, yellow urine, warmth and tenderness in the breasts or testicles, prostatitis, premenstrual irritability, and serious or intense menstrual bleeding.

Long-term Pitta imbalance may contribute to impaired vision or blindness, persistent hypertension, fibromyalgia, gout, inflammatory arthritis, bladder and kidney infections, hyperthyroidism, adrenal weakness, migraines, fainting, meningitis, encephalitis, chronic fatigue syndrome, autoimmune diseases, and multiple sclerosis.

In males, high Pitta can induce epididymis inflammation, inflammation of the prostate, and burning pain during ejaculation. In women, excess Pitta can cause inflammation of the endometrium and other reproductive tissues.

CHARACTERISTICS/ QUALITIES OF PITTA TYPE

Pitta type are well-structured, manage projects, and focus extremely well. They're willing to do something, and they're essentially predisposed. They are a treat as teachers, since their lessons are logically arranged, and everyone can obey their straightforward way of speaking.

The Pitta type spends money more systematically and more prudently. An open-plan office or working in a store will make life more difficult for him/her and colleagues to share the same space.

Pitta type loves to play outdoors and enjoy comparing their talents with others to prove their fighting spirit. They choose light, loose-fitting clothing made of natural fabrics, both in summer and in winter.

The qualities or characteristics of Pitta are oily, sharp, hot, light, fleshy, spreading and liquid, salty, sour, and pungent in taste. Therefore, choosing more of the attributes or characteristics of food and lifestyle choices that have the opposite effect, such as rough, dull, cold, heavy, static, stiff, dry, bitter, astringent, and sweet helps maintain equilibrium or bring balance to Pitta's excess.

People with Pitta-dominated Prakriti are medium build, with a reddish complexion, sun-sensitivity, industriousness, enthusiasm, and a strong appetite. They can be perfectionists, detail-oriented, and challenging. They usually don't like the hot weather. They sweat rather quickly and profusely. They tend to maintain a stable body weight irrespective of how much they consume. And they never skip meals because it makes them irritable and dysfunctional if they do.

They have a strong intellect, great metabolism, are beautiful, have glowing skin, sleep through the night, and have inner peace and happiness.

Alongside a moderate athletic physique, Pitta type gain weight equally or on the bottom half. They have smooth, lustrous, warm skin and they get warmed easily. They have a high metabolism, healthy appetite, and decent digestion.

Pitta type are driven, aggressive, creative, and highly intelligent, with a strong level of insight and prejudice. They like to be in charge and at the center of attention; they are highly focused innovators with energy levels that suit and can be likened to the 'Type A' personality. The Pitta type, though nocturnal, are deep sleepers and vulnerable to intense dreams and nightmares.

Pitta is Oily

Pitta's first attribute is oily (Sasneha or Snigdha in Sanskrit). The oily nature accounts for the softness of the skin, but in excess, it can also manifest itself as oily skin or acne. It can manifest as oily skin, oily hair, acne, excess mucus, or an especially cynical (think slippery) personality. Pitta people have a hard time tolerating oily foods and would do their best to minimize unhealthy, fried foods in their diet.

Otherwise, they may be prone to problems with their liver or gallbladder due to increased bile content, which is not properly assimilated in the body.

Pitta is Light

Light (Laghu) is another attribute of Pitta Dosha. It manifests itself differently from the light quality of Vata Dosha.

Pittas happen to be very prone to bright lights and sunshine. Lightness also expresses itself as a lean, fit physique, easy digestion, light-heartedness, a lively and aware mind, a charming or positive attitude, light-colored eyes, and fair skin. If in excess, it can induce stiffness, light-headedness, excess upward moving energy (think migraine or baldness), low blood sugar, or vulnerability to sunlight.

As a result, they are more vulnerable to moles, freckles, and melanoma than either Vata or Kapha. You are likely to wear glasses and need sunglasses during the day. Pitta people have strong appetites and can become hypoglycemic or light-headed if they don't eat on time or miss a meal.

Pitta is Sharp

The sharp quality can manifest itself as a sharp, bright intellect; or in abundance, as a sharp tongue.

Pitta people are very skilled, knowledgeable, and sensitive. They enjoy talking to other smart people. They do not waste their words and converse solely to learn or convey information.

A sharp mind is characteristically inquisitive, penetrating, fast, and very capable of mastery. Sharpness is also behind persistence, discernment, a powerful appetite, efficient digestive capability (which quickly breaks down consumed food), and bright vision—whether real, figurative, or both. In excess, it can lead to a quick temper, sharp tongue, the tendency to assess one and others unfairly, and strong hunger.

Pitta is Hot

Warm quality provides a nice blush in the cheeks, a naturally strong digestive flame, the desire to stay warm in cold conditions, and passion to the personality. "Hotness" may manifest as a warm, rosy skin, warm body temperature, and powerful metabolism and appetite; or, in excess, as ulcers, heartburn, or hot temper.

Like Vata people who feel cold easily, Pitta people tend to run hot (Ushna). They do not withstand heat well and choose to have cool environments and surroundings. Pitta people can be quite hot-tempered and easily lose their coolness. As Pitta imbalance occurs, they are also vulnerable to heartburn, inflammation, and ulcers. Eating hot, spicy food and drinking alcohol will aggravate Pitta Dosha.

Pitta Spreads

Being performance-oriented, Pitta people enjoy spreading (Saram) their name and popularity. This spreading quality can manifest itself as charisma and charm, as a capacity to transmit influence, and may contribute to outstanding accomplishment and popularity.

It can manifest as a tendency to spread name or influence an opinion around the local or global community. This quality is often behind a spreading rash and creating a toxic emotional environment.

Pitta is Liquid

The final quality of Pitta is liquid (Jala). Pitta type are susceptible to extreme thirst, sweat, and urination. Pitta is made up of fire and water components. Consuming too many liquids around or during meals impairs the fire and thus cuts out the digestive flame. Such quality can also express itself in the form of excess stomach acids.

Liquid quality encourages adequate salivation, good digestive juices, proper sweating, and fluidity of movement throughout the digestive tract, blood, joints, and body. However, excess liquidity can dilute the digestive flame, causing bleeding gums, bleeding problems in general, and a tendency to bruise easily. It can also manifest as excess sweating; when coupled with heat quality, it may appear as excess stomach acid.

Physical Characteristics

The first thing you notice with the Pitta-dominant people is their simplicity and their radiance. They are of average height, medium-sized eyes, and piercing glance; they are muscular and hungry for action.

Their skin is rather bright and sensitive, and the hair of the European Pitta type is often reddish or blond. Their gums tend to bleed, and their teeth are more yellowish than white. Their memory is accurate.

They sometimes have bright red hair, but baldness or thinning of hair is also popular in Pitta. They have a great metabolism, which sometimes leads them to believe that they can consume anything. They have a warm body temperature. They sleep soundly for short periods and have a strong sex drive.

When in harmony, Pittas has lustrous skin, great metabolism, plenty of stamina, and a good appetite. When out of control, Pittas can suffer from skin rashes, burning sensations, peptic ulcers, intense body heat, heartburn, and indigestion.

They are expected to have a well-proportioned skeletal frame that is medium in size, much like their overall bone structure and build. Their musculature is naturally lean yet muscular, and their weight is likely to remain fairly steady.

Their face is usually heart-shaped, and they may have distinct facial features such as a pointed nose and a tapered chin. The eyes are typically medium in size, light in color, and may be prone to bright light because the eyes are piercing.

(Please keep in mind that the differentiation between physical characteristics should always be recognized within the sense of ethnicity. For instance, traits such as eye color, skin color, or hair type are measured in contrast to others with common ancestry.)

Their skin and scalp are relatively fair, slightly oily, reddish in color, and may be particularly sensitive or reactive. Their hair is smooth and delicate, susceptible to early graying or balding, and may be either reddish or conspicuously red in color.

Their body temperature always seems to be steadily warm or hot, their extremities generally warm to the touch, and they sweat quickly. Thus, they are unable to withstand particularly hot weather, extreme heat, or intense physical work. They generally prefer to stay cold and prefer cooler, drier climates. Their inherent internal heat also makes them somewhat predisposed to inflammatory disorders.

Mental and Emotional Characteristics

Pittas have a strong mind and a great ability to concentrate. They're good decision-makers, coaches, and leaders when they're in harmony. They are precise, sharp-witted, straightforward, and often blunt. Out-of-balance Pittas may be short-tempered and argumentative.

They are generally intelligent and discerning—with excellent attention and memory, concise voice, and a mind as sharp, analytical, and reflective as it is concentrated and motivated. In fact, they almost undoubtedly love a good intellectual challenge.

They are known to be creative, hard-working, diligent, trustworthy, and smart, but they may also find like their iron will or their competitive nature dominates over the other facets of who they are.

In addition, Pitta type frequently ignore the needs of their bodies in order to fulfill their raw sense of motivation and their ability to be successful. They love learning and have a great ability to solve problems, systems, and managerial activities.

They are also likely to have a good sense of taste—in food and elsewhere in their lives—and while they are likely to make money easily, they can often waste it on luxuries. They tend to be highly principled, confident, and armed with natural leadership skills.

On the other side, they may have a bit of temper, and when their perfectionist tendencies take control, they may become highly critical of both themselves and others.

Pitta is full of energy, and those who belong to it are charming and charismatic, with a love of attention; in fact, it's a lot of fun to be around them as they're so lively and vibrant. They are also sharp-witted, competent speakers, and good decision-makers— particularly when they are in control. But when they are not, look out; they can be short-tempered, quickly frustrated, and argumentative.

In Balance

When healthy, Pitta provides contentment, easy digestion, good vision (light from the fire), brilliant intelligence, and glowing skin.

When we can think of Pitta in its balanced and unbalanced state, we can more easily recognize what it feels like when life comes into equilibrium, and quickly turn it around when we start moving away from it.

Pitta adds a lot of great things to our lives. It is the transformative power of our bodies and minds that turns food into nutrients and knowledge into comprehension. This is helpful in many ways, bringing in teamwork, strong leadership, and the capacity to absorb life experiences.

Mental absorption, sound judgment, and discernment are balanced Pitta features. The capacity to accurately sense what the body feels (sees, hears, smells, tastes, etc.) is controlled by Pitta.

Pitta regulates all the heat, digestion, and transformation of the mind and body. It regulates how we digest food, how we metabolize our sensory perceptions, and how we distinguish between right and wrong. Pitta is responsible for the essential digestive "Agni" or fire of the body. And when Pitta is healthy, our body functions at its finest; there are no health issues, especially digestion and transformation.

A balanced Pitta improves the capacity to follow goals and priorities via enhanced concentration, problem-solving skills, and trust.

When Pittas are in balance, they have a stunning combination of fire and water, which shows a strong, caring spirit, encouraging others to accomplish their goals. Pitta Dosha's unofficial mascot is a lion. They are powerful, energetic, demanding respect, and will defend their loved ones with fiercely loyal love.

Out of Balance

When out of balance, Pitta type can be controlling, emotional, judgmental, fiery-tempered, irritable, workaholic, overheated, and susceptible to rash and acne. They can suffer interrupted sleep, acid reflux, fatigue, and loose bowel movements.

When out of control particularly under the influence of alcohol, Pitta can become a furious, red-faced hothead. Pitta regulates the heat, digestion, and transformation of the body, mind, and soul. It regulates digestion, the processing of our sensory perceptions, and how we differentiate between things as correct or incorrect. Thus, the imbalance in the Pitta will lead to reduced digestion and also decrease the metabolism of the body. Ayurveda states that these two signs are the root cause of any other illness.

Pitta generally works on the gastrointestinal tract, liver, skin, eyes, and brain. The Pitta imbalance causes some or all of the following symptoms in the body which we discussed in the previous chapter.

What Causes Pitta Dosha?

Pitta Dosha appears to arise during the summer months, probably continuing through early autumn. Pitta may aggravate due to bad food choices, including over-intake of heating and spicy products, as well as over-intake of sour and citric fruits.

In addition, spending a large amount of time in hot conditions, such as in poorly ventilated kitchens or outside during peak sunshine, will increase Pitta that trigger imbalances.

Below are some factors responsible for Pitta Dosha:

• Unnecessary intake of pungent food. (Nearly all spices with a pungent, spicy taste raise Pitta Dosha.)

• Eating Pitta aggravating products. (pungent, sour, salty, very spicy, deep-fried, processed, red meat)

• Intake of caffeine (coffee), black tea, tobacco (smoking), alcohol, and other stimulants.

• Excessive ingestion of hot foods.

• Excessive intake of corrosive foods.

• Excessive ingestion of extreme-acting foods and drugs.

• Excessive frustration.

• Excessive fasting. (leads to an increase of digestion strength and thus leads to an increase of heat and excess Pitta Dosha)

• Prolonged sensitivity to sun radiation induces a rise in body heat and raises Pitta Dosha.

• Excessive sexual indulgence.

• Excessive consumption of sesame and sesame-prepared foods.

• Excessive consumption of flaxseed and flaxseed oil-prepared foods.

• Excessive consumption of curds—particularly when taste is sour.

• Excessive intake of fermented herbal beverages. (Induces an unnecessary rise in digestion fire and contributes to a spike in Pitta Dosha)

• Excessive intake of bitter and dried herbal beverages.

• Emotional tension.

• Overwork and/or poor rest.

Seasonal and Timely Causes

In the autumn season, Pitta Dosha normally rises in all people.

During the Summer Season:

In the afternoon: When we split the daytime into three sections, the middle one-third (10 am-2 pm) is occupied by Pitta.

Midnight: When we split the nighttime into three sections, the middle one-third (10 pm-2 am) is dominated by Pitta.

PITTA SUBTYPES/ SUBDOSHAS AND DISORDERS

W hile Pitta is a single entity, it has 5 subtypes, identified at 5 locations in the body. They are all interrelated, and the role of each Pitta depends on the functions of the others.

The 5 types of Pitta are:

• Pachaka Pitta—Located in the stomach and intestines

• Ranjaka Pitta—Located in the liver, spleen, stomach, and small intestine

• Sadhaka Pitta—Located in the brain/heart

• Alochaka Pitta—Located in the eyes

• Bhrajaka Pitta—Located in the skin

Subdoshas of Pitta points to the distribution of its roles. As described above, Pitta has its representations in 5 separate locations of the body. Such classification can be interpreted in terms of the functional distribution of Pitta.

Pitta subdoshas are ruled by Pachaka Pitta—the main and strongest Pitta subtype found in the digestive system, predominantly in the stomach and intestines. It governs all other Pitta subtypes by Agni Karma or fiery activity (promoting heat and energy). Therefore, the gut or Nabhi (Navel, the portrayal of the digestive system) is known to be the control station of all Pitta subtypes. This also means that much of the health, balance, and operation of Pitta subtypes is under the influence of Pachaka Pitta and therefore relies on the safety, balance, and action of Pachaka Pitta.

If there is an imbalance in the quality and quantity of Pachaka Pitta, the other Pittas would be affected, too. This leads to various disorders. For example, if Pachaka Pitta is functionally low (Manda Agni), the functions of other Pitta subtypes that are based on Pachaka Pitta would also deteriorate. If Pachaka Pitta is hyper (Ati Agni), the other Pitta subtypes often function in abundance and trigger systematic burnouts in a generic fashion or in their preliminary seats or locations.

Thus, Pachaka Pitta or central fire should be held in check with the utmost care and commitment.

But that doesn't mean that other subdoshas are not important. Each Pitta subtype has its own assigned roles—Pitta has its generic roles and operates at every corner of the body, regulating all functions. For example, if the task of obtaining and digesting food is delegated to Pachaka Pitta in the stomach, then the job to absorb the digested food and bring it into circulation and ensure that the food is properly assimilated and used at the cellular stage is assigned to other subdoshas.

Ranjaka Pitta gives color to the Ahara Rasa (digestive juices) flowing through the liver and spleen, making it crimson or bloody appearance, and thus taking part in the creation of Rakta or blood cells. Similarly, other subdoshas have their specific roles. The roles of all Pitta subtypes are synchronized—the integration of these Pitta subtypes is important to ensure that the activities of the body are smooth and uninterrupted.

Pitta subtypes also function in synchronization with Vata and Kapha subtypes for the preservation of a stable and disease-free atmosphere throughout the body. For example, in the digestion cycle, in the stomach and intestines, Pachaka Pitta works in coordination with Samana Vayu and Kledaka Kapha to enable proper digestion. Sadhaka Pitta works in sync with Tarpaka Kapha and Prana Vayu to enable a proper cycle of thinking to encourage knowledge and memory.

Pachaka Pitta

Location:

• The gastrointestinal tract along with digestive juice and certain enzymes (stomach, duodenum, and small intestine)

Action:

• Digestion of food and the differentiation between valuable components and waste parts of the food

Pitta that digests food and prepares it for further usage in the gastrointestinal tract is Pachaka Pitta. It is found in the stomach and small intestines.

Pachaka means it aids in digestion and metabolism in the body. This plays a part in breaking down food and extracting nutrients from the body. Compared to other Pitta subtypes, it has less Drava (liquid) content, but more Ushna (hot) content. It is also named Agni (digestive fire) in Ayurveda.

Pachaka accounts for hydrochloric acid, digestive enzymes, and pepsin, as well as intestinal digestive juices that are secreted from the small intestine villi. Pachaka Pitta deficiency typically results in hyperacidity, hypoglycemia, sugar cravings, gastritis, peptic ulcers, indigestion, anorexia, and dyspepsia.

It regulates digestive fire and the temperature of our body, retains the circulation of power, extracts nutrients from food, helps to create tissue, and has an anabolic effect. Pachaka also controls the temperature of the food, extracting the essence from the waste. The imbalance may contribute to slow or irregular digestion, heartburn, ulcers, or malabsorption.

Diseases Due to Its Aggravation:

Reduced Pachaka Pitta causes the following diseases:

• Reduction of appetite—it takes place due to reduced secretion of digestive juices and a complete decrease of all the quality of Pachaka Pitta

• Decreased hunger

• Indigestion

• Malabsorption

Increased Pachaka Pitta results in the following health conditions:

• **Appetite Deficiency:** It is triggered by decreased release of stomach acid, which induces lack of appetite, anorexia, heartburn, and gastritis. Throughout Ayurveda, it is called Pitta Agnimadhya. In this form of loss of appetite, the Drava (liquid) content of Pachaka Pitta is raised, but the Ushna (hot) level is decreased, resulting in malabsorption and loss of appetite.

• **Increased Appetite:** When Pachaka Pitta has a normal level of Drava (liquid) content, everything goes well. But when it's

Ushna (hot) and Tikshna (sharp) content is elevated, the individual feels an enhanced appetite and has a regular urge to eat and digest food very quickly compared to the normal individual.

Ranjaka Pitta

Location:

• Liver

• Spleen

• Stomach

• Small intestine

Action:

• Synthesis of hemoglobin

• Imparting red color to hemoglobin

Ranjaka Pitta is primarily found in the liver, small intestine, spleen, and stomach; it often exists in the blood and travels downwards. When the food is broken down by the Pachaka, the Ranjaka shapes it into the tissues, especially the blood. Toxins, whether attributable to contaminated food, water, and air or insufficient Pachaka activity can induce a specific imbalance in Ranjaka Pitta. Impaired Ranjaka may contribute to blood disorders like anemia, elevated or low cholesterol or blood pressure, and chronic fatigue syndrome.

Ranjaka Pitta provides color to blood, bile, skin, hair, eyes, urine, feces, saliva, and poop and also plays a major role in the temperature of blood in our circulatory system.

It is responsible for erythrogenesis, i.e. the production of red blood cells in the bone marrow. Ranjaka Pitta disintegrates hemoglobin in the liver to create heme and globin. This destroys bacteria and viruses in the spleen and creates certain white blood cells.

According to Ayurvedic doctors, "There is a mutual unity within the liver, stomach, spleen, and bone marrow." The activity of each of these organs has an impact on the other. The spleen is responsible for cleansing the blood and moving the leftover aged red blood cells into the liver. The liver kills the aged red blood cells and utilizes them to produce bile, pigments, and enzymes.

There is a correlation in Ayurveda between certain emotions and organs. For example, the liver is connected to rage, fear, anxiety, envy, hate, and jealousy. If such feelings are not understood and processed, they stay undigested or blocked, which may trigger inflammation in the liver to build up in the tissues which ultimately trigger diseases.

Diseases Due to Its Aggravation:

- Jaundice
- Hepatitis
- Chronic fatigue syndrome
- Mononucleosis
- Anemia
- Liver and spleen disorders

Sadhaka Pitta

Location:

• Heart

• Brain and nerves

Action:

• Metabolic activities in the brain

• Data processing and cognitive processes

• Maintaining the roles of the mind

• Sharper memory

Sadhaka is localized in the nervous system, especially in the brain and heart. It integrates ideas and perceptions and regulates thought, motivation, intellect, and self-esteem. It is therefore responsible for the metabolic operation of the brain and the transmission of information and cognitive processes.

Sadhaka Pitta is located in the grey matter of the brain as other neurotransmitters, and in the heart as a cardiac plexus or Heart Chakra. 'I' is essential for intelligence, empathy, sympathy, and appreciation; it is the location of the self, the "I am" which turns experiences into thoughts and emotions.

Sadhaka Pitta is our brain and heart link, which regulates the mental strength and mental assimilation ability of the nervous system and senses. This has an internal stream, so it's primarily located in the brain. Sadhaka Pitta controls our intellect, regulates our internal combustion, regulates the release of energy from our experiences, and gives us the power of bias; the absence of Sadhaka Pitta can create doubt.

Unbalanced Sadhaka can cause heart attack, unconsciousness, depression, or lack of appreciation and will. Many feelings, such as ego, intelligence, rage, happiness, commitment, fear, and determination are attributed to Sadhaka Pitta.

Diseases Due to Its Aggravation:

- Impairment of memory
- Deterioration of natural mental functions

Alochaka Pitta

Location:

- Eyes

Action:

- Vision is the primary feature of Alochaka Pitta. It detects the light and then sends it to the cortex.

The Pitta that allows seeing the light through the eyes is called Alochaka Pitta. The key location of the Alochaka Pitta is in the eye, which regulates the luster, color, and translucence of the eyes. It also regulates our visual perception and is also responsible for absorbing illumination. It plays a part in all our senses and our emotional reactions. About all eye disorders (except cataracts, for example) are the consequence of imbalanced Alochaka.

It maintains eyeball temperature, iris color, light sensitivity, sensory awareness, and three-dimensional sight. The deficiency in Alochaka Pitta results in short-sightedness, short-sightedness, conjunctivitis, stye, iritis, burning feeling in the eye, and light sensitivity. Metabolic behavior in the rods and cones of the retina is attributed to Alochaka Pitta.

Diseases Due to Its Aggravation:

• Eye defects or blurred vision

Bhrajaka Pitta

Location:

• Skin

Action:

• Color and texture of the skin

• Maintaining the warmth of the skin

• Digestion of natural medications applied externally to the skin

Bhrajaka Pitta is present in the skin and helps preserve the temperature, texture, color, and tone of the skin. It controls the warmth/heat through the skin; it can be referred to as the "Natural Glow." It handles perceptions of touch, temperature, and pain. Bhrajaka turns nurturing touch into healing and absorbs everything on the surface—sunlight, oil, or pollutants.

Abnormalities in Bhrajaka Pitta can result in skin conditions such as eczema, dermatitis, acne, anaesthesia, tingling, and numbness. Also, since the skin is connected to the liver and all internal organs, we accumulate unresolved anger, terror, and tension inside the connective tissue under the skin.

Diseases Due to Its Aggravation:

• Most skin diseases

Disorders

1. Sloughing blood

2. Sloughing of muscles

3. Burning feeling in the skin

4. Cracking of skin

5. Itching of skin

6. Burning Feeling

7. Scorching

8. Burning sensation

9. Boils

10. Acid reflux

11. Pyrosis (heartburn)

12. Internal burning sensation

13. Burning sensation in the shoulder

14. Excessive temperature

15. Blue spot

16. Herpes

17. Jaundice

18. Bitter taste in the mouth

19. A metallic odor from the mouth

20. Bad odor from the mouth

21. Excessive thirst

22. Dissatisfaction

23. Stomatitis

24. Pharyngitis

25. Conjunctivitis

26. Proctitis

27. Penis inflammation

28. Hemorrhage

29. Profuse sweating

30. Fetid body smell; unpleasant body odor

31. Cracking body ache

32. Urticaria

33. Red vesicle formation

34. Bleeding disorders

35. Red round patches

36. Fainting

37. Greenish or yellowish discoloration of the eyes, urine, or stools

DO YOU NEED TO BALANCE PITTA?

A nswer these questions to see if you're going to have to balance Pitta:

1. Do you feel pain and fatigue during hot weather?

2. Are you a perfectionist, or look for perfection in your stuff?

3. Do you get hot flashes?

4. Is your skin gritty and sensitive to acne and rashes?

5. Are you always frustrated or impatient?

6. Do you suffer from acidity often?

7. Are you having loose bowel movements?

8. Do you have a desire to be controlling or serious?

9. Are you often irritated, furious, or intense?

10. Is your hair started graying or thinning prematurely?

11. Do you wake up in the early hours and find it impossible to fall asleep again?

If you replied "YES" to any of these issues, you have to balance your Pitta Dosha.

MANAGING PITTA DOSHA

P eople with a pronounced Pitta Dosha are urged to live more reasonably, to maintain purity in thoughts and actions, and to select food, attitudes, habits, personal relationships, and environmental circumstances that could be instrumental in balancing Pitta characteristics.

Routine is a huge part of the Ayurvedic lifestyle, particularly if you're operating on Pitta—a dosha that will require the most continuity and stability! It helps to combat Pitta's natural tendencies and disorders.

So, here are some tips to help you build a simple, versatile, Pitta-balancing routine. These tips are not meant as a strict set of guidelines, but instead as a useful checklist for maintaining a sense of order that can be quickly enforced in your Pitta lifestyle. You can also notice smoother skin and a stronger sense of balance if you manage to follow this routine.

The Basics for Managing Pitta

The management of Pitta type can be summarized by "Moderation and Calmness." The very first thing that comes to mind while talking of Pitta is the ultimate blaze of fire. Pitta type are hot, fiery, oily, and intense. The management of Pitta type is therefore based on:

• Cooling

• Calming

• Moderation

Yoga is ideal for the Pitta type to let out steam, but the best yoga asanas are mild movements. It is necessary for people with a very prominent Pitta to prevent extremes. The same relates to food; here, in fact, very large quantities should be avoided.

It is beneficial to stay away from heat sources and try to search for a calm, well-ventilated environment. Feelings should be shared. Deep oil massage and meditation are both great.

Topics including Pitta pacifying foods, Pitta aggravating foods, essential herbs, oil massages, yoga asanas, and other important topics have a separate chapter for each. Here we'll just look at the basic lifestyle changes that you need to adapt...

Restore and Maintain Balance

As suggested for all three mind-body constitutions, priority should be given to life-management routines. And to have a good understanding of purpose, make sure you know why you're doing what you're doing. Be sure that you are living your life in relationship to the infinite.

Cultivate the mindset of becoming a valuable force for growth. Resist ego-fixing; cultivate serenity and mental calmness. Ignore mental attitudes, emotions, behaviors, and relations that activate and intensify Pitta (hot, fiery) characteristics.

Add Tastes that Favors (Prefer Sweet, Bitter, and Astringent Tastes)

It's perfect for a Pitta person to have fresh, cooling food. They have trouble skipping meals as they seem to have heavy appetites. Since they do have good digestive systems, they tend to handle raw foods better than the other doshas, but they must be careful to avoid hot foods, alcohol, caffeine, irritability, high aggression, and rage as they generate too much Pitta and disrupt the digestive system.

In addition to the key attributes of Pitta, it is also important to know certain tastes that raise Pitta and those that pacify it. Pungent, sour, and salty tastes aggravate Pitta by raising its hot quality. An example of a pungent taste is chilli pepper; of sour, pickles; and of salty, salt. Sweet, bitter, and astringent tastes can pacify Pitta by offering the opposite qualities of Pitta. An example of naturally sweet taste is wheat; of bitter and astringent (often combined), several leafy greens and herbs.

As the sweet, bitter, and astringent tastes decrease Pitta, these tastes should be prevalent in your diet. Remember that this is not necessarily a green light to consume processed sugary food and beverages. The naturally sweet flavor present in many grains, squashes, natural sweeteners, and fruits is most fitting and can help balance the Pitta. They all reduce Pitta influences; include them in your food plan. Complex carbs, milk, and some fruits are sweet; some green leafy vegetables are bitter; beans and some green vegetables are astringent.

Ahead in the book, there are separate chapters for each on what to eat, Pitta pacifying and non-pacifying foods, how to eat, and other essential tips.

Like Increases Like

Ayurveda's fundamental tenet is "Like Increases Like." Thus, growing Pitta's inherent qualities can increase Pitta in the body, mind, and soul.

For example, since Pitta is naturally hot, hot environment, hot food, hot seasons and times of day, and even hot emotions will increase Pitta. Likewise, the warm environments will enhance the quality of the liquid and therefore raise Pitta.

For example, if you're a Pitta type, and you hit the equator for a holiday and sunbathe for 6 hours a day and eat sweet, spicy food for one week daily. By the end of the week, you will have an intense rash and horrible heartburn, and you will find yourself in a bad mood. Ayurvedically, heat-increasing indulgences have raised the natural heat in your Pitta system and have contributed to the 'eruption' of hot conditions in your body and emotions.

Workouts are Must

And it has to be calm and mild. Yoga, tai-chi, cycling, swimming, biking, tennis, golf, and some other fun sport may be beneficial. But remember, exercise for fun and a feeling of well-being, don't be too competitive or aggressive.

Perform Cooling Activities

Do stuff that cools your mind, your feelings, and your body. Cultivate the values of integrity, justice, compassion, humility, self-control, constant learning, and thoughtful life, knowing that you collaborate for the betterment of humanity.

The perfect atmosphere for Pitta type is cool and dry. Cold weather activities like skiing and ice hockey, or early morning workouts are the best. Sweet scents, melodic songs, and gentle feelings are also good for Pittas.

Meditate Daily

One of the strongest Pitta remedies is to 'Surrender.' If you can build a gentle trust in—or relationship with—divine influence or natural force that you feel will do a fine job of orchestrating personal and spiritual life, it will relax your mind and take the weight off.

For this cause, it is helpful for a Pitta individual to have daily meditation. (And really enjoy it; don't just do it as if it's another task that you need to master). Meditation provides a break to the overheated Pitta. It soothes and relieves the mind. Be grateful, too, for what you have and what you have accomplished.

Balance Your Work Pace

Pittas must manage their activities and rest. Extended working hours and little to no rest will make matters worse. So, seek to strike a compromise between job time and rest time. Give your body and mind time to rest and unwind.

Be cautious of extended working hours and limited resting time, both of which are not healthy. Keeping a consistent daily schedule of 9 am to 6 pm, followed by 7-8 hours of sleep, is perfect for you.

Be with Nature

A 15-minute walk in the early morning or late evening is healthy for the body. Also, when you have time, you should go on a dive in the bay, a holiday on the hills, or anywhere you are surrounded by nature. It has the power to restore the body and mind.

Don't Skip Meals

Pitta can't do without food. You can feel like you may skip a meal, but never do it because it's not healthy for your digestive system. Maintain a regular meal schedule with breakfast, lunch, and dinner.

Be Joyful

Be happy and content. Sit down with your friends and relatives, share your emotions, love them, and laugh with them.

Go for Oil Massage (Abhyanga)

Massaging the body with warm oil or Pitta pacifying oil will be a relief to you. A gentle self-massage with warm coconut oil every day, 10–20 minutes, cools the intensity of Pitta and helps you to relax and 'go with the flow' rather than using your power to control the flow.

Ahead in the book, there is a separate chapter where you'll find the complete information on what oil to use, how to use, and other essential tips.

Yoga for Pitta Balance

Twisting, folding, wide-legged poses act as an appropriate challenge to fulfill the need for intense relaxation, while at the same time calming the body and strengthening the mind.

As a sister science of Ayurveda, yoga is an outstanding activity and philosophical practice to integrate into the everyday routine of maintaining the human constitution. While several yoga poses are helpful to any of the doshas, the key advantage in balancing your dosha is your approach and the way you perform your pose.

A Pitta individual's yoga practice will promote humility, tolerance, calm commitment, and relaxation in behavior.

Ahead in the book, there is a separate chapter where you'll find the complete list of essential yoga asanas, how to perform, and other essential tips.

Consume Herbs

Using herbs to manage your health complements the adjustments you bring to your food and lifestyle. Brahmi, Bhringaraj, and Guduchi are 3 major herbs used to extract excess Pitta from the body and preserve equilibrium.

Ahead in the book, there is a separate chapter where you'll find the complete list of herbs and other essential tips.

Wear Cool Clothing

Go for light and cool colors like purple, blue, pink, etc., particularly during summer. Pitta's favorite color is white.

Avoid Fumes

Seek not to go to areas where a lot of chemicals or fumes are emitted. The polluted locations are not nice for you, so stay away from them.

Be Emotionally Strong

A Pitta aggravated condition can make you emotionally weak. Too much stress will make you feel stressed, nervous, and sad. So, keep yourself at a moderate point. You can do so by expressing your feelings with your family and friends.

Extra Precautions

• Prevent ripped or over-sweet fruits.

• Avoid too much work or activity.

• Prevent too much stress.

• Avoid getting overly emotional.

• Avoid heavy foods such as fried foods, very spicy foods, and refined packaged items.

• Avoid too much coffee or tea.

• Resist alcohol or drugs.

• Maintain balance in all aspects and don't take yourself too seriously (Moderation is the key for Pittas).

• Go to bed by 10 pm.

• Be cautious not to overwork or strain your eyes with a screen or TV, particularly in the evening (get f.lux or any other software that gets rid of blue light).

• Take time to play, especially with children.

• Enjoy exercises like swimming, skiing, walking in nature by the water bodies, yoga, but avoid getting overheated or overburdened in competitive sports.

• Shield yourself from the mid-day sun (avoid heat).

• Take time to have a nutritious lunch (don't miss lunch).

• Enjoy cool—but not ice-cold—beverages.

• Food should be freshly cooked and slightly unctuous.

• First thing in the morning after brushing your teeth and rinsing your mouth, have some pure water left overnight in a cup of pure copper (It is extremely helpful in flushing toxins from the body).

PITTA DOSHA AND FASTING

asting is considered being an essential medicine in Ayurveda, as long as it is not a long-term fast that would deplete the individual. It is the traditional cure of nature for various diseases. Through expelling Ama (toxic buildup) from our digestive tract, fasting releases calming energies and boosts the immune system.

Pitta is fond of an occasional power trip. They like to eat a lot of food. Fasting for Pitta Dosha is a struggle because they have strong digestion. However, as the season switches, Pittas can fast.

Fasting Purposes

There are 3 aims of fasting:

• To provide optimum rest to the digestive system.

• Detoxifying the digestive tract and removing foreign materials.

• Restoring natural healthy digestion.

While zero fasting (no food at all) is not advised in Ayurveda since it will overstrain the power of Agni (digestive fire), the possibilities for your Prakriti fasting plan are still diverse and wide-ranging.

While for a lean person, vegetarian lunch and hot ginger tea for several weeks are adequate, others will require 3 meals a day, put together to provide optimum support for his or her purification. In the case of sensitive types, it might also be better to have just one soup day a week.

For most instances, people of the Vata and Pitta type should not fast for more than a day, as long-term fasting will increase the corresponding dosha in the body. Therefore, fasting is supposed to be performed cautiously.

Pitta individuals can fast on liquids—fruit (prune, grape, or pomegranate) or vegetable juices and broths—or on lightly cooked vegetables, but never on water alone. They should also never skip on quantity. Cucumber juice, which is both astringent and bitter in flavor, is another decent option and can avoid strong, sour-tasting juices.

Fasts can last 2-3 days, not more than that. And Pitta type are suggested to do fast only 4 times a year, as seasons shift. If you have a Vata-Pitta constitution, please add khichdi to your fast, or concentrate on grounding vegetable broths and fennel tea. Intermittent fasting is also ideal for Pittas.

In intermittent fasting, food should be consumed within the 8 hours window and no food should be consumed for the rest of 16 hours (The way I do this is I have my dinner at 7 pm and breakfast on the other day at 11 am).

The basic theory for the duration of fasting is as follows:

"Fasting starts when you no longer have the hunger; fasting stops when you experience the hunger and your body vigorously wants food."

Things to Remember When Considering Ayurveda and Intermittent Fasting

1. Select the duration of your fasting.

2. Eat a lot at lunchtime and a small quantity of food at breakfast and dinner.

3. Eat when you're hungry.

4. CCF (cumin, coriander, and fennel) tea is suggested for everyone.

5. If you have chosen to fast once a week, try to do so on a specific day.

6. Feeling sleepy or light-headed is a positive sign of fasting which will soon be over.

7. Meditation is also really relevant.

How to End a Fast?

When you're finished fasting, it's crucial not to rush back into the normal diet immediately. Doing so could cause your stomach upset. Upon completing an all-day juice fast, for example, you can have some fruit or a small amount of hot cereal for breakfast the next day, preceded by a plain, easy-to-digest lunch.

Here are a few tips to break the fast as per Ayurveda:

• Get a small amount of hot cereal for breakfast

• Pick a light and simple meal for lunch

It's necessary to take the same amount of time to prepare, fast, and get off the fast. Suppose, if you're planning a two-day pomegranate juice fast, you'd benefit from consuming a lighter, cleaner diet two days before you start, and then taking two days to gradually make your way back to your solid diet. Otherwise, you may worry that your digestive fire is doing more damage than good.

After a fast, it's not surprising to notice that you have fewer cravings and are automatically attracted to things that are healthier for you. After all, you will reap the rewards of fasting.

Precautions

1. Listen to your body.

2. Start slowly and gradually increase frequency.

3. Complete fasting (starving) is not recommended for our modern lifestyle as it will not burn fat and may actually induce weight gain (It increases Vata—the root cause of most diseases).

4. Proper nutrition of the body has to be maintained at all times.

5. Impulsive fasting can actually be detrimental to health.

6. Monitor your physical, emotional, and mental state before embarking on a fast.

7. Stop if feeling weak, depleted, irritated, or hungry.

8. Stop if experiencing symptoms such as a rash or headache.

9. Avoid all wheat, dairy, alcohol, meats, processed foods during a fast.

10. Eat light throughout the week to support the body and ensure maximum cleansing.

11. Monitor your appetite as you come out of the fast.

12. Metabolism slows down during a fast, thus going back to the daily eating routine gradually will avoid weight gain (especially for Kapha type).

When Not to Fast?

Fasting can be slightly depleting for those that are young, very elderly, pregnant, breastfeeding, menstruating, underweight or undernourished, or who have a chronic disease. So be sure to consult a professional Ayurvedic practitioner if you have a chronic problem or are on medication.

Also, while you plan to incorporate fasting into your healing regimen, note that Ayurveda is a deeply individualized method, and it is necessary to recognize and appreciate your own specific strengths and challenges. Over time, you can slowly intuit when you need to fast and when you need to relax your system.

Conclusion

As usual, there's no "one size fits all." It's about personalization, learning your dosha, and being mindful of what works and what not. Isn't that a wonderful thing? With that knowledge, whether or not you want to follow intermittent fasting, you can feel fantastic knowing that you choose to nurture and take care of yourself.

Pittas can fast, but usually, they don't like it because they have such large appetites. Nevertheless, for overeating Pittas, occasional fasting will help keep things under control. Intermittent fasting is best for them!

The only warning for Pittas is that fasting might raise the digestive fire (Agni) a little too much. So, if you continue to feel heated, aggravated, and irritable, it may be time to break

the fast.

PITTA AND COOLING FOODS

A yurveda considers the correct food and proper digestion to be at the core of good health. As per Ayurveda, fiery Pittas should consume foods with a cooling essence or nature.

Pittas have more fire than any other type; they're hot-headed. Hence, the sharp, hot nature of Pitta Dosha needs to be soothed by the cooling food. On the other hand, if we need to pacify the aggravated Pitta, it is better to avoid foods with hot and sharp properties such as ginger.

What does 'Cooling Foods' Mean?

Cooling foods are generally related to the temperature of the food. In Ayurveda, however, we also talk about the energetics of foods; whether food has cooling or warming properties. In the case of Pitta, it is best to have food filled with cooling and hydrating properties.

Cold neutralizes the hot and the hydrating properties neutralize the drying tendency when the fiery Pitta is out of balance. Some foods—coconut milk and spices like fennel seeds—can even make Pitta aggravating foods (like tomatoes) congenial to the Pitta Prakriti or Pitta body type. For example, the introduction of coconut milk to the spicy curry makes it digestible and assimilable to the individual of Pitta Prakriti without aggravating the Pitta, which can cause acidity.

Thus, eating more cooling foods, such as leafy vegetables abundant in bitter flavor, is a healthy way to balance Pitta. Sweet juicy fruits like pears can cool Pitta quickly. Spices that are not so pungent or hot including turmeric, cumin, coriander, cinnamon, cardamom, and fennel are recommended.

Pitta's body type also benefits from raw foods that tend to have a cooling quality, particularly during the spring-summer season. Conversely, it is better to limit the sensitivity to hot fiery meals (foods with a sharply warming energetic, alcohol, and caffeine); all of these will enhance internal heat and aggravate Pitta.

You should also take note of the spices you choose. Most of the spices are warm in nature, so pay particular attention to those that complement Pitta. Consider cooking with soothing spices such as fennel, mint, and coriander, and reduce hot spices such as dried ginger and mustard seeds. (*You'll find a detailed list of Pitta-Pacifying Foods ahead in the book.*)

Raw foods are naturally cooling, and Pittas are able to manage them better than the other doshas; thus, adding in a variety of raw fruits and vegetables would usually be supportive— especially in warmer mo

nths.

Drink lots of room-temperature or cold water and drink 2-3 cups of Organic Pitta Tea (the recipe is ahead) during the day. Organic Pitta Tea includes soothing spices and rose petals, renowned in Ayurveda for calming the mind, body, and emotions.

Fresh fruit juices and coconut water are perfect pick-me-ups on warm days of summer. At bedtime, mix some organic rose petal spread in the milk that has been boiled and cooled for a calming drink. Rose Petal Lassi makes a nice beverage for lunch.

Some Precautions to Keep

Although hot foods are not recommended for Pitta, be mind that it is not healthy to eat food that is fully cooled or is chilled. That is, don't have breakfast or lunch fully cooled off! The cooling food discussed here is connected to the cooling nature, not to the temperature.

Many foods that do not look hot and sharp to taste can still make Pitta worse if eaten in excess—fish and nuts. Such foods have a quality called 'Potency' which is hot. This makes Pitta worse. On the other hand, fennel seeds, when chewed, offer a sharp taste in the mouth, but because of its cooling potency, pacify Pitta.

One more factor to consider is that eating foods with cold properties such as cold milk-based drinks do pacify aggravated Pitta, however, when consumed in abundance for a long period, the optimal Pitta level is disturbed. This optimum level of Pitta is needed to support digestion. So be cautious not to overeat these cooling foods.

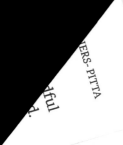

TASTES THAT PACIFY PITTA

O ne of the basic teachings of the Ayurvedic tradition is that everything in the universe consists of 5 elements— earth, water, fire, air, and ether (space). The tastes are no different; each of them contains all 5 elements. That said, each taste is made up of 2 elements.

The 6 Tastes and Their Predominant Elements:

Sweet (Madhura):	Earth and Water
Sour (Amla):	Earth and Fire
Salty (Lavana):	Water and Fire
Pungent (Katu):	Fire and Air
Bitter (Tikta):	Air and Ether
Astringent (Kashaya):	Air and Earth

How Tastes Influence Doshas?

The 6 tastes help balance our doshas with what we're consuming. Sweet taste, for example, creates earthy Kapha, cools hot Pitta, and reduces airy Vata. Because it is a nourishing taste, it increases the volume of all tissues. Therefore, we live off sweet-tasting foods—oats, root vegetables, and rice—because they keep us healthy and strong. There are 3 ways in which tastes influence the doshas. They are:

Temperature

Each taste often affects the body's temperature, either by heating it up or cooling it down. Like, cinnamon is pungent and warm, which increases body temperatures. Grapes are sweet and cooling, which can help you cool down.

Quality (Heavy or Light, Wet or Dry, Penetrating or Soft)

Taste defines the quality of whether food is light or heavy to digest, or wet or dry on mucous membranes. Black pepper is spicy, light, dry, and penetrating—easy to digest, dries mucous membranes, and penetrates deeply into the tissues. Chew on the peppercorn and these characteristics will be obvious to you!

Direction (Where the Food Goes in the Body)

Remarkably, the tastes have an affinity to certain parts of the body. Like garlic goes to our lungs as we can smell it. Ginger has multiple 'sites' like clearing mucus from the lungs, heating the skin, stimulating the blood, and relaxing the muscles. Asparagus is known for having the smell of urine—Ayurveda says asparagus is a bitter, cooling food that releases internal heat through the urinary system.

It's no accident that we use these 6 tastes to define emotional experiences or patterns quite explicitly. We equate love, kindness, and caring nature with sweetness. We have a mutual understanding of what a salty individual's personality could look like, and most of us can evaluate someone who has become particularly bitter over the years.

Remember, Ayurveda views taste—from the most tangible sensory experience to the subtlest energetic influence—as an essential therapeutic tool. While each of the 6 tastes has a vital role to play, the perfect combination of tastes can vary widely from one person to the other.

Pitta is primarily composed of fire and water elements, which make Pitta light, sharp, hot, oily, liquid, spreading, and subtle. Because of these characteristics, Pitta is balanced by the sweet, bitter, and astringent tastes and aggravated by the sour, salty, and pungent tastes.

Below, you'll find a deeper understanding of how each taste specifically affects Pitta, as well as how you can balance Pitta by emphasizing certain tastes and minimize certain tastes.

So, to balance Pitta:

Emphasize

Sweet

The sweet taste is made up of water and earth and is perfect for balancing Pitta. Of the 6 tastes, sweet is considered to be the most calming and nourishing. It encourages durability, energy, and healthy body fluids and tissues when consumed in moderation.

If you're looking to add weight, it's a good taste to emphasize. It's heavy, oily, and moist attributes in slow digestion.

The sweet flavor is abundant in products such as wheat, rice, dairy, cereals, dates, pumpkins, maple syrup, and liquorice root.

• Having the sweet taste does NOT require us to consume huge quantities of refined sugar or sugary sweet food; naturally sweet food is much better.

• Pursue naturally sweet foods such as sweet fruits, most grains, squash, root vegetables, milk, ghee, and fresh yogurt.

• The sweet flavor is soothing and heavy, but still anti-inflammatory. It soothes heat, reduces thirst, benefits skin and hair, and appears to be grounding, nourishing, sturdy, and satisfying.

Bitter

The bitter taste is made up of air and space. It's known to be the coolest and lightest of all tastes. Thanks to its cooling properties, it is extremely detoxifying and can help extract toxic material from the body. Bitter food always tends to purify your mind by liberating you from desires and addictive feelings. It's best for Pittas!

• The bitter taste is prominent in bitter greens—like kale, dandelion greens, and collard greens. It is also present in bitter melon, Jerusalem artichokes, dark chocolate, and Pitta pacifying spices such as cumin, neem leaves, saffron, and turmeric.

• The bitter taste is exceptionally cool but also drying.

• Bitters clean the pallet and enhance the sensation of taste. They condition the skin and muscles, protect the circulation, alleviate burning and scratching feelings, ease hunger, control the appetite, encourage digestion, and help to reduce heat, sweat, and excess Pitta.

Astringent

The astringent taste is made of air and earth. It's cool, dry, and firm. Most beans and legumes are astringent and may induce gas, which is why Vatas should consume astringent taste in moderation. Pitta benefits most of the astringent taste's coolness, and its dry, light qualities balance Kapha. Like bitter food, astringent food tends to purify and strengthen the skin.

Unripe bananas, green grapes, pomegranates, cranberries, green beans, alfalfa, and okra are all astringent foods.

• The astringent taste is simply a dry flavor—a chalky taste that dries the mouth and can cause it to contract (picture biting a raw green banana).

• The astringent taste is heavy, cold, and dry.

• Pittas benefit from the compressive, consuming, union-promoting aspect of the astringent taste. This may reduce the tendency of Pitta to aggravate, tone the body tissues, avoid bleeding disorders, thwart diarrhea, and even remove excess sweat and fluid.

Minimize

Pungent

• Pungent is a hot, spicy taste contained in chillies, radishes, turnips, raw onions, and others (especially hot spices).

• It is especially hot and light—both characteristics that disrupt the Pitta.

• Too much pungent may cause excess thirst, burning sensations, bleeding, dizziness, and inflammation (especially in the intestinal tract).

Sour

• Limit sour foods such as vinegar and other processed foods, hard cheeses, sour cream, green grapes, pineapple, grapefruit, and alcohol (Occasionally, beer or white wine is ok though).

• Pitta is exacerbated by the hot, light, and oily taste of the sour foods.

• Too much sour taste may raise thirst, interrupt circulation, trigger muscle pain, trigger pus in wounds, and create burning feelings in the throat, chest, or heart. Also, negative emotions like resentment or envy may be encouraged.

• The occasional squeezing of the cooling lime juice as a garnish is the perfect way for Pitta to get a sour taste.

Salty

• The salty flavor is perhaps entirely derived from the salt itself.

• Like the sour taste, it is salt's light, dry, and oily essence that makes Pitta worse.

• Salt taste can disrupt the balance of the blood, inhibit sensory organs, increase fire, worsen the skin, increase inflammation, trigger tissue breakup, trigger water retention, high blood pressure, intestinal inflammation, gray hair, wrinkles, and excess thirst. It can also increase our desire for stronger flavors, which can trigger Pitta far more.

SPECIFIC PITTA
PACIFYING FOODS

When you've been advised to work on managing Pitta, one of the greatest things you can do is to add Pitta-pacifying foods to your diet. Pitta is supplemented by a diet of fresh, whole foods (both cooked and raw) that are cool, nutritious, energizing, fairly dry, and high in carbohydrates.

These foods soothe Pitta by lowering internal heat, preventing inflammation, calming the digestive fire, grounding the body, and absorbing excess fluid and oil. Since Pitta is of a relatively substantial sort, an adequate diet is a very effective way of encouraging a balance.

The intense, hot nature of Pitta Dosha needs to be calmed by soothing food. The best Pitta foods are generously warm with fairly thick textures—i.e. not steaming hot food.

You can put the oily nature of Pitta to harmony with the aid of dry food in your everyday diet. Including some heavy foods will supply your fast-burning constitution with strength and steady nourishment.

Take cool, refreshing food in summer, such as salads, milk, cold water, and ice cream (in moderation). Herbal tea, specifically mint or liquorice root teas, pacifies Pitta. Cold oats, cinnamon bread, and apple tea is a perfect Pitta breakfast. Vegetarian diets, in general, are the best for Pittas, since the intake of red meat continues to heat the body from fat. Milk, grain, and vegetables are also beneficial.

Below is the specific list of food items that you can take into account to pacify Pitta rapidly:

Fruits

Fruits that pacify Pitta are usually sweet and quite astringent. Dry fruits are usually appropriate but are only good in limited amounts, so as not to further exacerbate Pitta's tendency for rapid digestion.

Fruit and fruit juices are better eaten alone—30 minutes before, and preferably at least 1 hour after all other meals. It tends to ensure optimum digestion.

Note:

1. Fruits should be sweet and ripe; eliminate fruits that are sour or unripe. Also avoid green grapes, oranges, pineapples, and plums until they are sweet and ripe.

2. This rule does not apply to fruit that we normally consider vegetables (avocados, cucumbers, tomatoes, etc.). You'll find these in the "vegetables" category.

Favor

- Figs
- Pears
- Watermelon
- Pineapple
- Melons
- Plums
- Applesauce
- Pomegranates
- Prunes

- Raisins
- Strawberries
- Grapes (red, purple, black)
- Limes
- Mangos
- Apples
- Apricots
- Berries
- Cherries
- Coconut
- Dates
- Oranges
- Papaya

Vegetables

Vegetables that pacify Pitta would usually be a little sweet and either bitter, astringent, or both. Many vegetables have a mixture of these tastes, so playing with a broad range of vegetables is a perfect way to diversify your Pitta pacifying diet.

Pitta will typically digest raw vegetables faster than Vata and Kapha, but midday is often the best time of day to have them since the digestive power is at its maximum.

Favor

- Artichoke
- Rutabaga
- Spaghetti
- Squash
- Leeks (cooked)
- Sprouts (not spicy)
- Squash (summer)
- Squash (winter)

- Avocado
- Spinach (raw)
- Sweet Potatoes
- Watercress
- Parsley
- Wheat Grass
- Zucchini
- Asparagus
- Collard Greens
- Cucumber
- Dandelion Greens
- Green Beans
- Jerusalem Artichoke
- Celery
- Bell Peppers
- Cilantro
- Kale
- Leafy Greens
- Mushrooms
- Parsnips
- Olives (black)
- Lettuce
- Onions (cooked)
- Peas
- Brussels Sprouts
- Pumpkin
- Radishes (cooked)
- Beets (cooked)
- Carrots (cooked)
- Peppers (sweet)
- Potatoes
- Cauliflower
- Bitter Melon
- Okra
- Broccoli
- Cabbage

Grains

Grains that pacify Pitta are cooling, sweet, dry, and grounding. Grains appear to be staples in our diets and, overall; Pitta benefits from its sweet, nourishing nature. You may also note that many of the grains that benefit Pitta are quite dry; this tends to accounts for the oily nature of Pitta.

Favor

- Barley
- Quinoa
- Rice (basmati, white, wild)
- Sprouted Wheat Bread
- Rice Cakes
- Seitan
- Amaranth
- Spelt
- Tapioca
- Wheat
- Durham Flour
- Granola
- Couscous
- Oat Bran
- Pancakes
- Pasta
- Wheat Bran
- Cereal (dry)
- Oats
- Crackers

Legumes

Legumes are usually astringent in taste and are also mostly Pitta-pacifying. So, feel free to enjoy a wide variety of them.

Favor

- Adzuki Beans
- Black Beans
- Mung Dal
- Black-Eyed Peas
- Garbanzo Beans (Chickpeas)
- Kidney Beans
- White Beans
- Soy Beans
- Tofu
- Lentils
- Lima Beans
- Mung Beans
- Navy Beans
- Pinto Beans
- Split Peas
- Soy flour
- Tempeh

Dairy

Dairy goods are soothing, nourishing, and refreshing, and many of them are Pitta pacifying.

Favor

- Yogurt (homemade, diluted, without fruit)
- Cottage Cheese

- Cow's Milk
- Ghee
- Butter (unsalted)
- Cheese (soft, unsalted, not aged)
- Goat's Cheese (soft, unsalted)
- Ice Cream
- Goat's Milk

Nuts and Seeds

Nuts and seeds are highly oily and are typically warm, but most of them are not great for Pitta. That said, there are a few types of nuts and a few seeds that are suitable in limited quantities; they are less oily and are either slightly warm or cool in nature.

Favor

- Pumpkin Seeds
- Almonds (soaked and peeled)
- Charoli Nuts
- Popcorn (buttered, without salt)
- Flax Seeds
- Sunflower Seeds
- Coconut

Meat and Eggs

Pitta goes best with animal foods that taste sweet, are fairly dry (like rabbits or venison), and are either moderately warm or cool in nature.

Favor

- Venison
- Eggs (white only)
- Buffalo
- Chicken (white)
- Fish (freshwater)
- Rabbit
- Turkey (white)
- Shrimp

(However, as per Ayurveda, non-vegetarian foods are never suggested! As per Ayurveda, we are energy beings, so when we consume meat, we're introducing the pain, fear, guilt, and all other negative emotions related to that meat that took place during the death of it. As a result, it accumulates negative energy in our body. Ayurveda always recommends a fresh and healthy vegetarian or vegan diet.)

Oils

Besides being oily in nature, Pitta works well with a small amount of oil—as long as it cools. The perfect Pitta oils are sunflower oil, ghee, coconut oil, and olive oil.

Favor

- Coconut Oil
- Flax Seed Oil
- Primrose Oil
- Sunflower Oil
- Soy Oil
- Walnut Oil
- Ghee
- Olive Oil

Sweeteners

In general, naturally occurring sweet tastes are much more balanced than processed sugary sweets, meaning that even the best sweeteners should be used in moderation.

Favor

- Barley Malt
- Turbinado
- Date Sugar
- Fructose
- Maple Syrup
- Rice Syrup
- Fruit Juice Concentrates
- Sucanat

Spices

Some spices are usually warm and thus have the ability to aggravate Pitta. The spices to be chosen should only be slightly warm, helping to sustain a healthy digestive fire without inducing Pitta and, in some cases, deliberately cooling.

In particular, the calming properties of cardamom, cilantro, coriander, fennel, and mint tend to relax the heat of Pitta. On occasion, such spices can be used to render foods that may otherwise be too hot for Pitta to tolerable. Cumin, saffron, and turmeric—even though are warm—also provide some valuable Pitta pacifying properties.

Favor

- Basil (fresh)
- Fennel
- Spearmint
- Tarragon
- Coriander (seeds or powder)
- Turmeric
- Vanilla
- Ginger (fresh)
- Mint
- Black Pepper (small amounts)
- Neem Leaves
- Orange Peel
- Cumin (seeds or powder)
- Parsley
- Peppermint
- Cardamom
- Wintergreen
- Cinnamon (small amounts)
- Dill
- Saffron

Drinks

They are best taken at room temperature or cooled (mildly warm is also good).

Favor

- Herbal Teas (with bitter and astringent taste—alfalfa, chicory, dandelion, hibiscus, and strawberry leaf)
- Milk
- Wheatgrass Juice

- Pitta Tea (available online or in your nearest tea shop)
- 'Chai' or Black Tea (in moderation)
- Fruit Juice (diluted with one-half water; in moderation)

NON-SUGGESTED MEALS

Attempt to reduce warm, oily, and light food. Below is the list of food items that should be moderated for Pitta's balance:

Note: You should avoid consuming these food items daily, but occasionally, you can have them.

Fruits

Fruits to be avoided are those that are particularly warm or sour (like bananas, cranberries, and green grapes). You can see several fruits both in Favor and Avoid columns below, since different types of the same fruit may be pacifying or aggravating, based on how sweet or sour they are. When attempting to balance Pitta, learning to differentiate between these tastes and preferring sweet fruits over sour ones is always beneficial.

Avoid

- Grapefruit
- Apples (sour)
- Pineapple (sour)
- Apricots (sour)
- Mangos (green)
- Oranges (sour)
- Peaches
- Bananas
- Berries (sour)

- Cherries (sour)
- Tamarind
- Grapes (green)
- Kiwi
- Lemons
- Persimmons
- Plums (sour)
- Cranberries

Vegetables

The only veggies to minimize or eliminate for Pitta are those that are particularly spicy, hot, sharp, or sour—garlic, green chillies, radishes, onion, and mustard greens.

Avoid

- Peppers (hot)
- Radishes (raw)
- Daikon
- Turnips
- Radish
- Eggplant
- Beets (raw)
- Turnip Greens
- Onions (raw)
- Burdock Root
- Corn (fresh)
- Garlic
- Beet Greens
- Green Chillies
- Horseradish
- Kohlrabi
- Leeks (raw)

- Mustard Greens
- Olives (green)
- Spinach (cooked)
- Tomatoes

Grains

When it comes to managing Pitta, avoiding warm grains such as buckwheat, corn, millet, brown rice, and yeast is the most important.

Avoid

- Buckwheat
- Corn
- Muesli
- Rice (brown)
- Rye
- Yeasted bread
- Millet
- Polenta

Legumes

Beans that are not ideal for Pitta are those that are especially sour, oily, or heating.

Avoid

- Miso
- Urad Dal

Dairy

Those to avoid are sour, salty, or hot. Dairy milk (cow's milk, goat's milk, sheep's milk, etc.) should be consumed at least one hour before or after any other meal.

Stop consuming milk with meat for this reason. Almond and rice milk are fine alternatives if you choose to mix milk with other foods or if you cannot digest milk easily.

Avoid

- Buttermilk
- Cheese (hard)
- Yogurt (frozen, store-bought, or with fruit)
- Butter (salted)
- Sour Cream

Nuts and Seeds

Nuts and seeds are highly oily and are typically heating,;most of them are not terrifically balancing for Pitta.

Avoid

- Almonds (with skin)
- Brazil Nuts
- Pistachios
- Tahini
- Cashews
- Pine Nuts
- Chia Seeds
- Filberts
- Macadamia Nuts
- Peanuts

- Walnut
- Pecans

Meat and Eggs

Meats that do not work are those that are especially oily, salty, or heating (dark chicken, beef, salmon, tuna).

Avoid

- Salmon
- Chicken (dark)
- Lamb
- Duck
- Eggs (yolk)
- Fish (saltwater)
- Beef
- Pork
- Seafood
- Tuna Fish
- Turkey (dark)
- Sardines

Oils

The quality of Pitta is hot and wet, it is therefore treated with cooling, sweet oils that are heat dispelling, drying, healthy, and soothing. Here are certain oils that Pitta type should be avoiding.

Avoid

- Safflower Oil

- Almond Oil
- Corn Oil
- Sesame Oil
- Apricot Oil

Sweeteners

Since the sweet taste soothes Pitta, most sweeteners are well tolerated by Pitta, but some are simply too warm or processed for Pitta.

Avoid

- Honey
- White Sugar
- Jaggery
- Molasses

Spices

For Pitta, the food should be spiced mildly to moderate and never really hot or cold. The overall spiciness is more important than the individual spices when spiced.

Avoid

- Garlic (raw)
- Ginger (dry)
- Horseradish
- Marjoram
- Nutmeg
- Oregano

- Anise
- Asafetida
- Calamus
- Sage
- Cayenne Pepper
- Hyssop
- Poppy Seeds
- Star Anise
- Thyme
- Mustard Seeds

Drinks

Though Pittas can enjoy most beverages, avoid consuming large quantities of any of them. Plus, you should strictly avoid the following drinks.

Avoid

- Alcohol
- Sweet Fruit Juices
- Tomato Juice
- Soft Drinks
- Carbonated Water
- Coffee
- Spicy Herbal Teas

HOW TO EAT FOR PITTA BALANCING?

Y ou can have Pitta disorders even after an optimum Pitta diet. The reason could be the wrong eating patterns.

Some key ways to balance the doshas are by what we consume and drink every day, and just as important how and when. Ayurveda really considers the correct diet and proper digestion to be at the root of good health.

When it comes to pacifying Pitta, how we eat can be just as important as what we eat, and this is a particularly useful topic to focus on if the possibility of radically changing the diet is overwhelming right now.

Pitta is profoundly soothed when we eat in a quiet environment —one where we can devote our full attention to the process of being nourished.

Routine itself also controls Pitta, and the practice of consuming three square meals a day (at the same time every day) also decreases Pitta and helps to improve weak digestion.

As we have already discussed, the aggravating properties of many Pitta-aggravating foods can be reduced by ensuring that they are cool, sweet, ripe, and generously garnished with butter, ghee, and certain digestive spices in moderate quantity. But also visualizing your meal—which is grounding your energy, nourishing your body, and fostering health and wellness through good eating habits—will go a long way towards pacifying Pitta.

Suggested Meals

Pre-Breakfast

The perfect way to start the day is to have a cup of mint refresh tea with peppermint leaves, roses, coriander seeds, hibiscus flowers, fennel seeds, and liquorice; or Pitta tea with ghee, or honey and turmeric.

Breakfast

While lunch is known to be the most crucial meal of the day, a nutritious breakfast helps to maintain the energy levels balanced in the morning.

Normally, breakfast is not to be missed when Pitta is aggravated. There is a wide range of balanced breakfast foods to choose from. Workable options are those that are sweet, high in carbohydrates, and still deliver sustainable energy.

• A perfect breakfast may be as easy as a date and an almond shake made from soaked dates, soaked and peeled almonds, and boiled milk (or a substitute)—mixed with cardamom and a pinch of cinnamon.

• A delicious fruit salad (apples, pears, red grapes, and blueberries) garnished with raisins and shredded coconut. This lighter meal is definitely going to fit best in the warmer months than at the end of winter.

• Oatmeal or rice porridge mixed with hot milk and flavored with raisins or chopped dates, sliced almonds (soaked and peeled), ghee, and maple syrup is another one you can go for.

• One more is wheat or barley cream, or rice or wheat with coconut milk and ghee. This may be garnished with spices such as cilantro and coriander, as well as crushed nuts such as almonds.

Lunch

Ayurveda finds lunch to be the most essential meal of the day, implying it's the biggest and the most nutritious. So no matter how crazy the schedules may be, consider a nutritious and balanced lunch that involves a range of food groups.

Ideal foods for lunch includes basmati rice, split yellow moong dal, ghee, leafy greens such as broccoli and lettuce, bell peppers, radish, and mushrooms. You can garnish the meal with spices and herbs such as coriander, black pepper, turmeric, basil, and mint.

You may also look for whole-grain tortillas or pasta as an alternative to rice. A small portion of vegetable salad is also a nice option on the side and you may use dressings such as mint mayonnaise or sunflower oil.

Try something like:

• Red lentils made with soothing herbs such as cilantro, mint or fennel, buttered whole-grain bread (use unsalted butter), sautéed purple cabbage, and a green salad. Add vegetables such as carrots, celery, and onion to the soup. With ghee, sauté the cabbage with cumin, coriander, turmeric, lime juice, and a tablespoon of maple syrup.

• Seasoned tofu and steamed collard greens over wild rice. In sunflower oil, sauté the tofu and stir in some of your favorite Pitta pacifying spices. Garnish with olive oil, freshly squeezed lime juice, ground coriander, and black pepper.

• Whole wheat spaghetti, pesto, and fresh vegetables (bell

peppers, broccoli, carrots, celery, green beans, mushrooms, zucchini, or black olives). Garnish with minced chèvre, olive oil, and cilantro. Serve with some green salad and soup.

• Avocado fried rice and sprouted wheat bread with ghee or unsalted oil is another good option.

Dinner

Dinner for Pitta type can be a little smaller and lighter than lunch, but it still requires sustaining Pitta's healthy metabolism. A basic yet nourishing meal or a slightly smaller serving of lunch can do well. Your dinner can involve soup or broth with vegetables such as artichoke, cauliflower, and garbanzo beans.

If you're not up for soup, or if you want something more substantial, a whole grain pasta with identical vegetables will fit. One of the healthiest choices will be a khichdi bowl (a typical Indian dish that includes rice, cooked with chopped vegetables, and spices such as black mustard, cumin, cinnamon, fennel, coriander, and fenugreek seeds).

Individuals suffering from celiac disease or gluten sensitivity can use quinoa as a replacement for rice. This super-food is also widely promoted by dieticians thanks to its excellent nutritious content, not to mention its tasty nutty taste. You can also try adding parsnips, potatoes, carrots, and leafy greens, among others, to widen the variety of vegetables in your meals. Follow the meal with a glass of buttermilk or Lassi.

Other options are:

• Red mung beans with dill, combined with roasted asparagus and basmati rice.

• Veggie burgers with sautéed mushrooms, goat cheese, lettuce, avocado, and homemade fries.

• Double spiced rice, omitting mustard seeds and adding

cashews with soaked and peeled almonds, pumpkin seeds, or sunflower seeds and served with flatbread.

Snacks

Stick to sweet fruits, thus restricting the consumption of others with a bitter taste like most citric fruits. Fruits with a sweet or bitter taste make excellent snacks as they're Pitta-pacifying. Some good options include apples, pears, papayas, pineapples, and pomegranates.

Dry fruits, nuts, and seeds are also good snacking choices, but you need to stick with healthier varieties such as coconuts, flaxseeds, pumpkin seeds, and almonds.

It will also be a good idea to cool any evening snacks with a glass of cool milk, garnished with ghee and turmeric.

Some Other Important Factors

Quantity of Food

Ayurveda gives value not only to quality but also to quantity. Eat tiny quantities of food at regular intervals instead of big meals in one sitting. This is especially beneficial for your digestion because it will fulfil all the stages of your digestion.

Dining Environment

Sit down to eat in a quiet place and eat slowly, chew the food properly (ideally 32 times). Eating while walking, working, and talking is likely to trigger gas, indigestion, and acidity that Vata-Pitta type are susceptible to. Liquids should be taken one hour before or after the meal so as not to dilute the digestive juices. A couple of sips while you're eating are still fine, though.

Cook with Balance

It is often difficult to prevent all Pitta aggravating food. If that is the case, simply cook in Pitta pacifying mediums or mix them with the right Pitta pacifying food and spices. Use sweet tastes to help digest them properly without aggravating Pitta.

Timing Your Meals

As a Pitta type, you are probably already aware of the significance of a routine or 'Dinacharya.' Meal timings are an integral aspect of a routine and should be adhered to as far as possible.

You should have your:

• Breakfast at around 7:30-8:30 am

• Lunch at 12-2 pm

• Dinner between 7-8 pm

Obviously, adhering strictly to this schedule can be difficult, particularly when it comes to dinner time, but try not to delay it as much as possible.

So, cultivate an eating routine like your sleeping routine; the digestion will always benefit from a routine. Pre-program the meal times of the day so that you have the time to take charge of managing yourself.

Water and food are just next to the air for survival. Once the digestion is conditioned to kick in at certain fixed times by daily practice, it functions effectively to produce more Ojas out of the food you consume. Ojas is the most complex component of the digestive process—a biochemical material that sustains life and well-being. Nutrients from the food you consume are absorbed and assimilated to the fullest degree by your body, and the waste is filtered out quickly, leaving no room for 'Ama'— digestive toxins—to build up in your bloodstream and function as a breeding ground for imbalances and diseases.

Healthy Preparation and Serving of Food

• Make your food with love and care. It's all linked.

• For the food to be consumed to become Ojas, you have to prepare it with patience, a good attitude, care, and affection. Many cultures hold holy acts of cooking and eating. In the Vedic practice, the chef bathes and gives thanks to Agni (fire) before beginning the task of preparing the first meal of the day for the family.

• Must not cook food (or eat) while you are irritated or stressed since the liver and appetite are negatively impacted by stressful thoughts and cannot effectively digest the meal.

• Eat at a place or room designated for eating, not in front of the T. V. or at the workspace.

• Diffuse a pleasant mix of aromas in your dining area about an hour before you eat.

• Eating lemon, coriander, sweet orange and mint are healthy options for the stomach and the release of digestive juices.

• Make sure all you need for your meal is at your fingertips as you settle down to eat so that you don't have to get up or be distracted from your food once you start eating.

• Practice mindful eating. Multitasking while eating is a commonly seen habit that is sure to trigger various health issues that might be prevented if one only took the time to give the meal the attention it needs. The time that is considered as lost when solely eating doing nothing will provide improved vitality and productivity that the relished, well-digested food will provide.

• It's better to feed in quiet, with all the senses concentrated on the aromas, spices, colors, and textures of your food.

• Arguments, intensely stressful debates, and discipline with children are behaviors that are not suited to mealtimes.

Other Mindful Eating Habits to Follow

• Don't work or talk on the phone while you're eating.

• Don't read or watch TV.

• Offer thanks or sit down in silence for a minute before you start eating.

• Do not chew down the food; savor every bite and chew properly before swallowing.

• A few sips of warm water during the meal will aid digestion but do not consume too much of any drink.

• At any meal, avoid eating until you are very full. The perfect Ayurvedic portion is what you could hold with your both palms joined together. Leaving a space in your stomach after you're finished boosts digestion.

• Once you've finished eating, sit still for a couple of minutes; don't try to perform the next task of the day instantly.

Closing Words

Your diet is special, and these recommendations are intended to act as a guide. You can use your own judgment to select the best diet and mealtimes, although these Ayurvedic guidelines will also steer you in the right direction. Just make it a point to include as many Pitta-pacifying foods as possible using the information given.

After all, Ayurveda stresses the value of a healthy diet, and the entire variety of food accessible to humans is more than I can fit in this book! Simply stop eating highly processed and refined products, since these products are believed to raise the amount of 'Ama' and increase the likelihood of chronic lifestyle diseases.

PITTA SEASONAL GUIDE (RITUCHARYA)

A yurveda divides the year into 3 seasons, centered on the dominant basic forces or doshas conveyed in each season. The three doshas exhibit varying amounts of the 5 elements (space, air, fire, water, and earth). Optimal well-being occurs while doshas are in equilibrium, a state called 'Sattva.'

Each season is identified with a dosha in Ayurveda—Spring with Kapha, Summer with Pitta, and Autumn and Winter with Vata. Each of these doshas has a propensity to increase with the metabolism during its season. Thus, the heat of summer tends to make Pitta worse in us, while dry, cold, and windy winters tend to increase Vata.

Such seasonal variations of the doshas within us can be controlled by eating well for the season. Desh (place) and Kala (time) are important considerations when it comes to choosing what you eat. If you suspect, some of these choices come naturally to most of us—like we're heading for cool drinks on a hot day, and we're eager to wrap our fingers around a steaming cup of soup on a chilly evening.

Pitta dominates the summer, reigning from July through October in most parts of the Northern hemisphere. Summer is a season full of delicious food and drink—think of chips, salsa, and margaritas! However, several of these typical summer party foods can leave you with a Pitta imbalances like annoyance, excess body heat, and digestive problems. Also, for those with less Pitta, it is important to take measures to keep Pitta in control during this timeframe because of its seasonal effects.

Some symptoms of aggravated Pitta include jaundice, hepatitis, acute fatigue syndrome, mononucleosis, anemia, and liver and spleen disorders.

So, How to Reduce Pitta Dosha during Summer?

Avoid Foods that Heat You Up

When your body is hot, the last thing you need to do is rev it up with spicy food. Thus, go gentle with curries, chillies, spicy peppers, and salsas. Sour foods such as yogurt, cheese, and sour cream bring so much heat to the Pittas.

Too many hot, oily, fried, acidic, spicy, salty, sour, and fermented foods may make Pitta worse, as can coffee, alcohol, and red meat. Even onions, garlic, and nightshades like tomatoes, bell peppers, and potatoes are difficult for Pitta to digest, especially when it's hot and humid outside.

Instead, prefer the summer harvest. Enjoy cool and soothing fruits and vegetables, leafy greens, bitter and astringent sprouts, brussels sprouts, broccoli and cauliflower, and almost every grain.

Also, restrict too much salty food—it can leave you dehydrated and make your skin worse. Limited doses of ginger, black pepper, and cumin are all right but say no to cayenne. Stay away from tomatoes, onions, garlic, beets, and spinach whenever you can. Alcohol also has a heating effect on the body.

Favor Foods that Cool You Down

Sweet, bitter, astringent food are the right ones to go. Excellent sources are milk (drink it warm), butter, and ghee. Olive oil, sunflower oil, and coconut oil are perfect for calming Pitta.

Sweet, ripe fruits such as avocados, cherries, plums, oranges, pineapples, peaches, and mangoes are great. Cilantro and mint are excellent, and a little cinnamon is all right. Asparagus, cucumbers, sweet potatoes, broccoli, green leafy vegetables, zucchini, and green beans are all healthy.

Avoid Ice-Cold Drinks

"What, no ice in my drink? Isn't that the ultimate heat balancer?" No! Although we need to keep it cool, it's much more important to keep our digestion strong. Your digestive system is like a fire responsible for turning food into energy.

When the fires of your digestive fire burn in a balanced way, you will assimilate all the good bits that you need from your diet while removing the not-so-good bits. However, when you drink the iced-water at noon, you essentially put out the flames of your digestive fire. So lay off the ice and head to room temperature drinks. It'll be assimilated into your system quicker and you're going to be rehydrated faster.

Eat at the Right Time

An essential aspect of maintaining Pitta and holding things calm is to consume your main meal in the middle of the day when the digestive fire is strongest. Skipping meals is also a sure way to upset Pitta; note how cranky you feel when you skip lunch.

Exercise the Right Way

Exercising in a way that is too intense, too sharp, and heating may make Pitta worse. An approach is to relocate the workout to the cooler setting. If you prefer working out, do so at the time of the day when nature is coolest. That's best during the early morning. The second best is in the evening.

Light movement is advised, such as yoga, tai chi, walking, and swimming. Start the practice with more difficult poses and end up with relaxing and soothing poses, including wide-legged and wide-arm poses to expel heat from the groin and armpits. You may also cool down with pranayamas like Sitali and Nadi Shodhan.

Make Time to Play

When Pitta is out of balance, we seem to be demanding, aggressive, restless, and overdoing. It, in effect, produces further conflict. So, get this over with some downtime for fun. Allow yourself the time to play. Balance the intensity of the heat in your work with some fun 'Play-time.'

Soothe Your Mind

As the mind is, so is the body. The most effective way to relax the mind is to cultivate a regular meditation practice. There are, however, plenty of other ways to turn the dial down on the busy, frizzy mind. Listen to some lovely songs, try walking in nature, or do some mindful breathing to soothe the mind and the soul.

Relax Your Lifestyle

If your lifestyle is too stressful and on-the-go, you have a lot of tension and many responsibilities, and not a lot of relaxation time (i.e., excessive Vata); all these can increase the Pitta fire.

The Solution: Slow down, set aside quiet time, and offer priority to self-care. Take a non-working lunch and enjoy a nutritious meal—which encourages healthy nutrition in the body and mind. Switch off the stereo in your vehicle or leave your earbuds at home while you're on a walk or a run.

Take a holiday where you would be going to enjoy activities like surfing or spending hours in the shade. Perform some stargazing stuff; staring at the deep indigo night sky in the cool fresh air is a profoundly meditative experience. And don't feel like you have to say yes to every social invitation and job obligation—take some time for yourself!

Daily Summer Rituals for Pitta

1. Begin and end the day with a relaxing massage of the feet with oil such as sesame or virgin coconut oil. It'll help draw the heat down and out of the body.

2. Consider making herbal tea and then allow it to cool down. Finally, enjoy long, soothing, and refreshing beverages throughout the day.

3. Keep your food cool, light, and fresh, also seek to moderate spices.

Lifestyle Adjustments

The most valuable thing you can do for yourself is to keep yourself calm, physically and emotionally. Plan to go out during the cooler hours of the day, in the early morning or the evening —especially in summer. Shade yourself and consume lots of soothing beverages like peppermint tea or lime water and maybe some unrefined cane sugar.

Exercise early in the morning and seek not to push too hard. Integrate several twists and forward bends into your yoga practice, eliminate inversions, and try Sheetali Pranayama— a soothing breath. Also, cultivate a feeling of playfulness and relaxation to smooth the Pitta Sharpness.

PITTA BALANCING YOGA POSES

Yoga is the sister science of Ayurveda. Ayurveda is the healing side of Yoga; Yoga is the spiritual side of Ayurveda. Both combined are responsible for maintaining a healthy and balanced diet that fits your individual needs, investing in self-care rituals that sustain your body, mind, and spirit, and practicing asanas in a manner that is taught by this ancient science of life. These 3 components are your keys to good health and well-being.

The teachings of Ayurveda and Yoga have been given to us to work hand-in-hand. Understanding how the three doshas work in your body will help you to adjust to the changes that result from changes in your diet, how you live, and the surrounding environment. This knowledge is meant to guide you through your practice in yoga so that you can experience your best, both on and off the mat.

How are Yoga and Ayurveda Connected?

Yoga and Ayurveda are two paths that are intertwined in such close relationships that it is hard to imagine going down one of these paths without the knowledge of the other.

Ayurveda, which means "Knowledge of Life," is the ancient art and science of keeping the mind and body balanced and healthy. Yoga is the ancient art and science of preparing the mind and body for the eventual liberation and enlightenment of the soul.

Ayurveda tells us how to keep the physical body healthy and yoga tells us how this well-being contributes to our spiritual journey. Both Yoga and Ayurveda derive from ancient Sanskrit scriptures called the Vedas.

"Yoga is the practical side of Vedic instruction, while Ayurveda is the soothing hand." In fact, these approaches intersect.

In fact, Ayurveda and Yoga are so closely related that some people argue that the first codifier of Yoga and Chakra, the first codifier of Ayurveda, may have been the same individual. Philosophically, both Yoga and Ayurveda are based in Samkhya, 1 of the 6 branches of Indian classical thought.

What Sort of Yoga is Right for You?

For deciding the kind of yoga practice that is appropriate for you, the most important factor is your Vikriti or imbalance.

Your Vikriti is, in essence, the single most important determinant of your entire regime. Once you've fixed the mismatch, you will stay in good health by finding a yoga practice that fits your philosophy or lifestyle (It is sometimes complicated for a layperson to differentiate between traits that are inborn or natural and those that arise from excess. For best results, contact a qualified Ayurvedic physician).

People with a Vata nature or disorder are most helped by a yoga practice that is soothing, calming, and yet warming. People of Pitta disposition or disorder are most helped by a yoga practice that is soothing, calming, and cooling. And Kapha type are most helped by a yoga practice that is stimulating and warming. Each person has different needs. Practicing in a manner that does not help you is asking for a greater imbalance.

The Pitta-centered yoga practice is concentrated and somewhat challenging. After all, transformation always happens in the fire! However, the Pitta-focused practice may also be quite depleting due to increased physical and/or mental demands. People of all constitutions may be "burned out" by an excess of Pitta.

To balance the excess Pitta, we need to bring opposing 'Gunas' into practice—cool, dry, dull, gentle, and dark. And combining these 'Gunas' can begin with your approach to the practice—try to practice in a colder, darker environment with a more relaxed attitude (without aspirations, rivalry, or judgment).

The key locations of Pitta in the body are the small intestine, liver, and navel region, so emphasis should be on the navel and solar plexus. According to the concepts of Ayurveda, asanas that open up these areas can release heat and stress and help to alleviate Pitta. Therefore, backbends are great for Pitta— Bhujangasana (cobra), Matsyasana (fish)—as well as side bends and twists.

Calming poses serve to soothe Pitta's intensity and relieve the feelings of rage and frustration that Pittas are susceptible to. Through alleviating Pitta, these asanas are beneficial for disorders such as ulcers and hyperacidity, liver disorder, and acne. They also have a direct effect on the liver and spleen and help to control the intensity of the digestive fire.

Now, you might be wondering, 'Do I have to join a yoga class?' Well, not! Yoga can be easily done at home. All you need is a designated space (doesn't have to be much bigger than your mat), a regular practice period, and a determination to be consistent. Even if you haven't taken any yoga classes, you can easily learn how to conduct your home practice in a way that keeps Pitta relaxed and balanced.

Tips to Calm Pitta through Yoga Asanas

Yoga practice for a Pitta adult should be one that produces comfort, serenity, and nourishment. Pittas can cultivate this by following some basic guidelines:

• Have fun doing the poses. Don't take your pose or yourself too seriously.

• Love the flow of the poses.

• Soften your eyes down, on the horizon, or just practice with your eyes closed.

• Allow freedom and creativity in the practice.

• Spice things up. Stop sticking to a single style or sequence of poses.

• Train in a relatively comfortable place. You don't want to get cold, but Pittas should avoid practicing in highly warm environments.

• Focus on the feeling of yoga in your body, not your brain.

• Work with 80% effort.

• Avoid being judgmental and skeptical of yourself.

• Make sure you've got plenty of practice space.

• Note that yoga is not a competition.

• Focus on the exhalation.

• Use exhalation to let out any rage, irritation, pain, etc. that has been building up.

• Be mindful of the breath in your back body.

• Do a lot of bends and side body openings.

• Notice the position of your ribs; draw them back to your body.

• Benefit from practice at a moderate pace.

• Remember that less is more!

The Best Asanas for Pitta Balance

Stretching asanas is prescribed for all doshas and should be included in every warm-up routine. However, depending on the specific requirements of Pitta type, certain behaviors should be included in the routine. The list below provides you with information about your Prakriti yoga asanas.

The poses shown below are Pitta-pacifying that can be done individually or in sequence:

Ustrasana (Camel Pose)

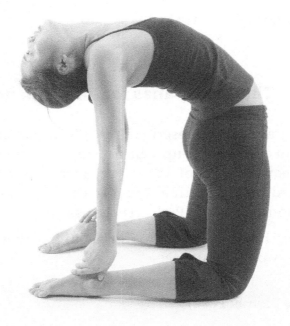

Ustrasana is really helpful to Pittas. This asana opens up the abdomen, the solar plexus, and the chest, enabling the free flow of energy across these areas.

Kneel with the butt raised as though you were standing on your knees. Place your hands on your buttocks. Shift your thighs and pelvis forward while you extend your lower back, taking your hands near your heels. Kindly stretch your neck out. Remember to breathe.

Uttana Shishosana (Puppy Pose)

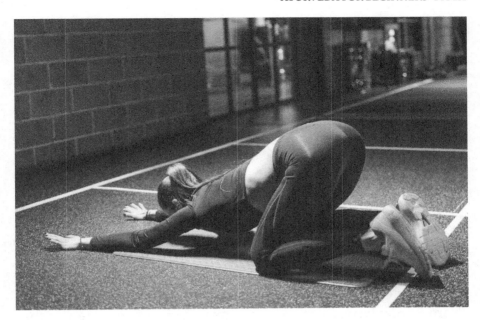

Start in the table-top position. The shoulders stack over the wrists, the hips stack over the knees, and the spine neutral. Inhale, move your hands forward as comfortably as possible. Exhale; melt the chest in the direction of the mat. Hold your hips raised and positioned straight above your knees. Hands stay shoulder-width apart.

Breathe deeply, feel the opening through the back of the heart space. Keep the pose for 4-6 breaths or longer if needed.

Adho Mukha Svanasana (Downward-Facing Dog)

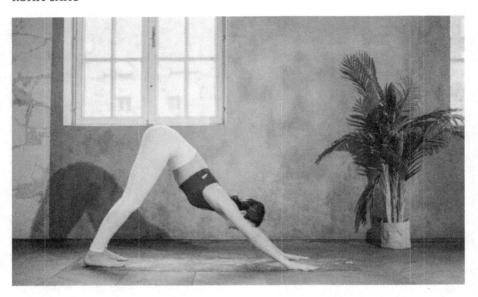

From Puppy Pose, move your hands in front of you a few inches and tuck your toes beneath. Inhale, lift your knees and press your hips up to create an inverted V-shape with your body. Exhale, push the heels to the ground and relax the heart space. Stay wide through the shoulder blades, spreading them on the back body. Keep the pose for 4-6 breaths.

Breathe deeply, soften, and relax into the posture. Release and pause before moving on to the next posture.

Janu Sirsasana (Head-to-Knee Pose)

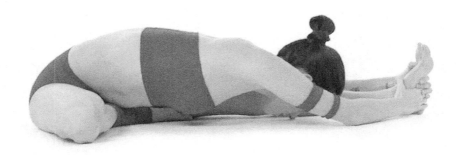

Sitting on your butt, extend your legs forward. Bend your left foot to rest against your upper right thigh, forming a "4" formation with your legs. Inhale; lift your arms upward. Exhale and move forward to your toes without bending the knee of your straight leg.

If you can't hold your foot, put your hands on your ankle, shin, or knee. Fold over your extended leg, keeping your back straight, but bowing your head towards your lower body. Take long, steady, deep breaths and keep the pose for 1-3 minutes. Switch the legs. Sit down, breathe, and relax before you move on.

Viparita Shalabhasana (Superman Pose)

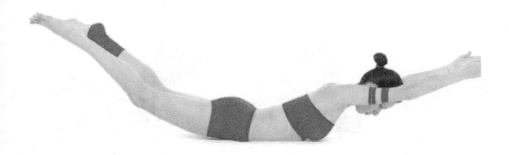

Lay flat on your stomach. While keeping all four limbs on the floor, spread out your arms and legs as if you were attempting to reach the walls in front of and behind you. Inhale and simultaneously raise your arms and legs off the ground, attempting to balance your pelvis and lower abs—but only get to a position where you can breathe easily. Relax the body in this elevated position and keep it for at least 20 seconds; release.

Bhujangasana (Cobra Pose)

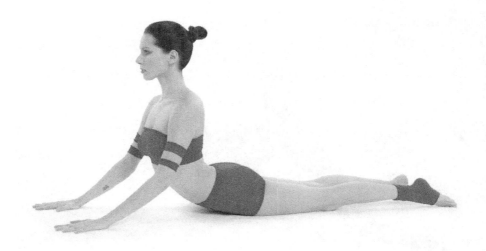

Start by lying down on the front body, the legs stretch long and the tops of the legs rest on the mat. The hands frame the chest while the elbows remain close to the ribcage. Push on the tops of the legs and the pelvis.

Inhale; press your hands to lift the chest off the ground. Exhale; draw your shoulders back and bring your heart forward. The shoulders remain away from the ears and the neck. Stay in this pose for as long as you like.

Prasarita Paddottanasana (Wide-Legged Forward Fold)

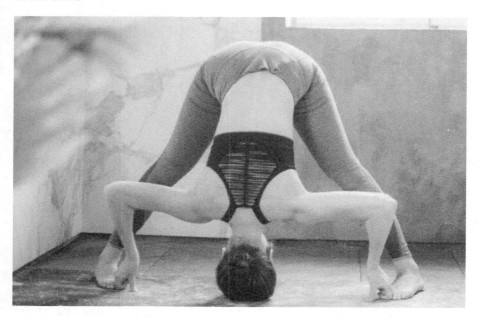

Stand longitudinally on the mat with your feet broader than the hip-width, as wide as you can comfort the body. Let your hands rest on the feet. Inhale; lengthen the spine. Exhale; gradually fold to the hips and release your hands to the mat or block.

Enjoy the fold for 5-7 breaths.

Ardha Hanumanasana (Runner's Lunge Twist)

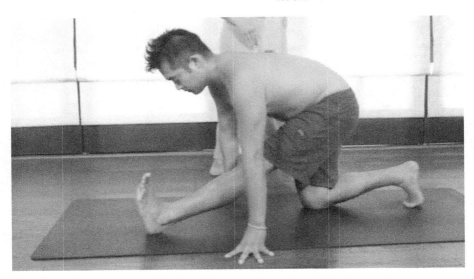

From a wide leg fold, bend to the left knee and pivot to face the short end of the mat in the lunge position of the runner. The right leg is straight—the ball of the foot is grounded and the heel of the foot is lifted. Place your right hand firmly on the ground.

Inhale; put the left arm in the air, the palm faced away from you. Exhale; twist the chest and torso to the left. The right leg remains straight and solid. Return to the runner's lunge after a few breaths in the twist.

Paschimottanasana (Seated Forward Fold)

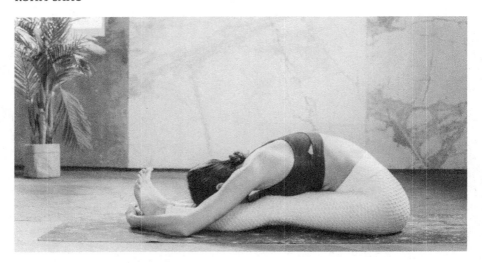

Paschimottanasana is grounding and allows you to release tension and heat through your feet, legs, and head.

For this, sit with both your legs stretched in front of you. Inhale; raise your arms and draw your spine high, engage your abdominal muscles slightly. Exhale; curl over the legs. Hold the torso lengthened and add a deeper curve in the knees if the hamstrings are tight.

Don't worry about touching your toes; let go of the temptation to overexert or push yourself to your limits. Allow the pose to wash over you like a cool, soothing ocean wave as you breathe. Hang on for 2-10 minutes.

Ardha Matsyendrāsana (Half Lord of the Fishes)

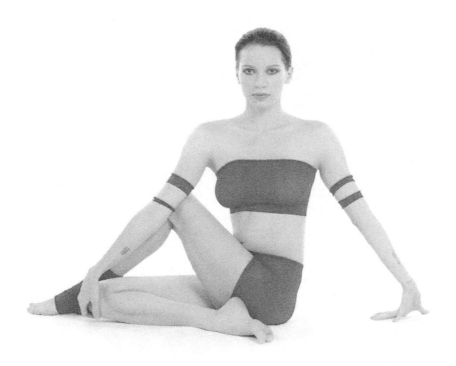

Bend your right knee and draw your leg towards you. From there, cross the right foot over the ball of the foot to the outside of the left hip. Inhale; raise your arms and lengthen your spine.

Exhale; rotate the torso to the right. Lay your left arm on your leg and place your right hand on the floor behind you.

Keep going through the spine while breathing deeply in the pose. With every exhalation, surrender yourself more to the pose and maybe deepen the twist. Release the twist after a few breaths and repeat on the other side.

Salamba Sarvangasana (Half Shoulder Stand)

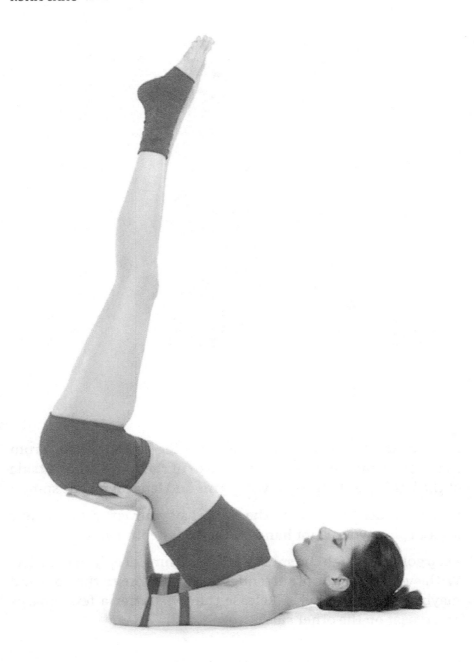

Lie flat on you back. Inhale to get ready. Exhale; press down through your palms, draw your knees in and lift your legs.

Find the position of the legs where they can balance and relax somewhat. Straighten the legs and put the palms of the hands on the lower back, holding the elbows close. Bear minimum weight on the head and neck and do not move the neck at all.

Keep the position for 6-8 breaths. To leave the pose, bend your knees to your forehead and roll your spine back to the mat very gradually, finally releasing your hands from your lower back.

Sarvangasana (Shoulder Stand)

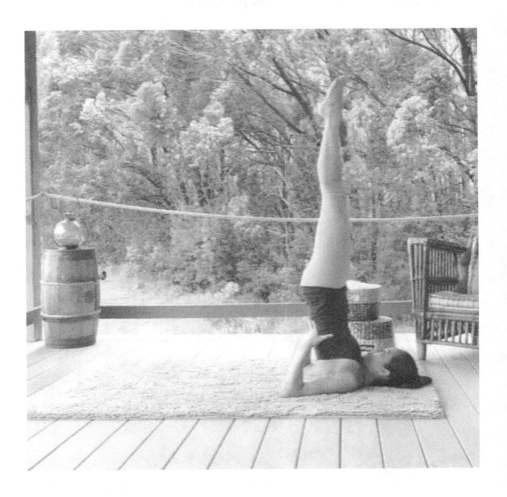

Not only does the Shoulder Stand have the cooling effect that all inversions do, but it also calms the agitated mind, which is so often the case when Pitta is too much.

As you hold the Shoulder Stand, let your mind fall to the ground. Imagine that all the emotions are emptying out of the brain and into the earth.

Let go and relax here for as long as you feel relaxed.

Viparita Karani (Legs Up the Wall Pose)

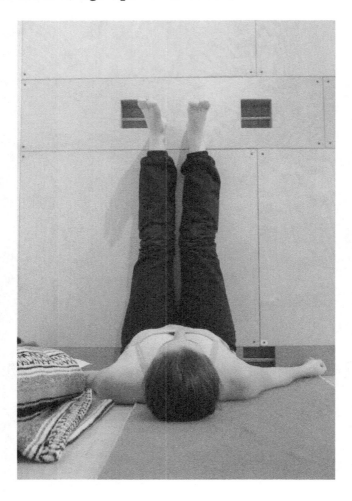

It's an alternative to Sarvangasana (Shoulder Stand). If you think that Shoulder Stand isn't safe for your body, consider Legs Up The Wall Pose instead.

If you don't have time to do all the postures on this list, this is the one pose you might do if you've got 5-10 minutes to practice. It's very effective for soothing the mind and the body. It doesn't require a lot of (if any) effort since the wall automatically supports the legs.

As you relax and breathe in this posture, carry with you the purpose of softening all aspects of your body and mind. The purpose is everything, so if you plan to do something during this pose, it can add much more impact to the body than simply doing a posture without intention.

Anjaneyasana (Pitta Low Lunge)

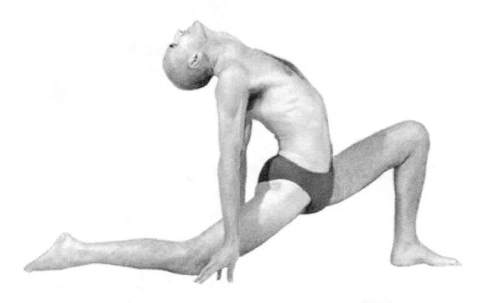

This is a unique Low Lunge version that also focuses on releasing energy downstream.

Enter the Low Lunge and take your hands to the floor or the inside of the front foot. Soften your shoulders down, gently push the top of your back foot into the ground, and lower your chin to your chest. You'll feel a release in the Psoas... that's all right, just don't push it!

Stay here for the next 4-10 breaths.

Ardha Chandrasana (Half-Moon Pose)

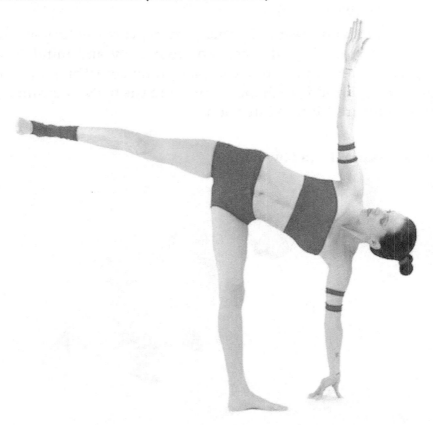

Now is your opportunity to expand and stretch. The aim is to feel flexible by keeping both legs engaged (buoyant, not constricted).

Enter the Half Moon with one or both hands on a block (if you need support). When you place both hands down, make sure you lift the hip of the raised leg up to the sky without straining the lower back. Concentrate on spreading the energy across the elevated leg and foot.

Hold your breathing steady and deep, and draw your navel in and out (Uddiyana Bandha) for support and a little lightness. Try this one for 4 breaths. Resist doing more. (Moderation keeps Pitta from doing crazy things!)

Sirsasana (Headstand)

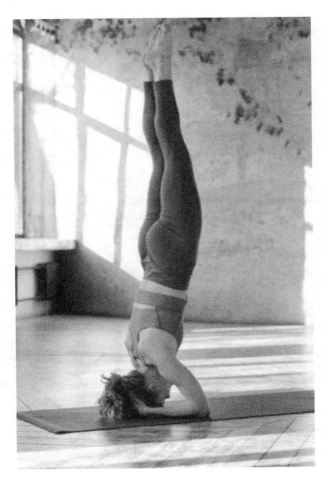

Headstands for people with Pitta imbalances can be avoided as they heat up the body and a lot of the heat accumulates in the head and eyes. The eyes are mainly a Pitta-controlled organ. For this reason, Headstands can cause or worsen eye diseases. So if you have any eye disorders, Legs Up The Wall Pose can be a great option for you.

But if you choose to do a Headstand, it can be kept for a very short period of time.

Baddha Konasana (Butterfly Pose)

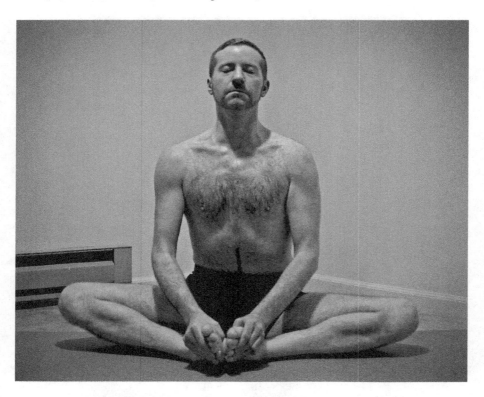

It is extremely cooling in nature. Butterfly Pose is ideal for the overly competitive Pitta because it's gentle and calming. Ease your way into a forward fold, but only fold as much as feels good for your body.

For it, come to a seated position and bring the soles of your feet together. Keep your spine tall and abs pulled in tight. Grab hold of each foot with your hands and place elbows against your inner thighs. Keeping your spine long, inhale to prepare, and as you exhale, slowing lower your torso forward pausing when you feel the stretch. Hold for 30 seconds or more.

There's no need to push it. Always pay attention to the sensations that arise rather than pushing through any kind of pain or discomfort.

Marjaryasana (Cat-Cow Pose)

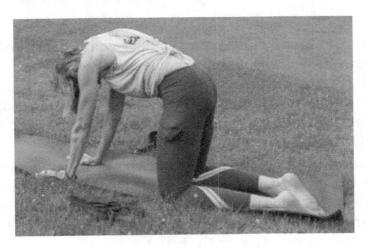

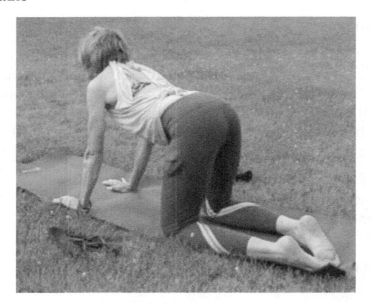

To perform, keep your hands shoulder-width apart and your knees directly below your hips. Inhale deeply while curving your lower back and bringing your head up, tilting your pelvis up like a "cow." Exhale deeply and bring your abdomen in, arching your spine and bringing your head and pelvis down like a "cat." Repeat several times.

Make sure to synchronize your breath with your movement. Inhale like that of an arch, and exhale like a round. These postures are claimed to help spread and regulate the fire energies throughout the body (It is said that when Pitta becomes out of control, fire accumulates in the belly).

Picture the fires in your belly spreading through the rest of your body. Since yoga is all about movement with attention and intent, it's always a good idea to use a little visualization during a pose.

Garbhasana (Child's Pose)

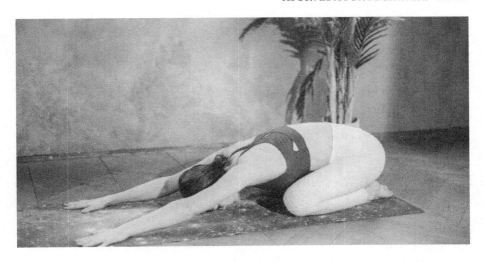

Child's Pose is an inherently relaxing and soothing posture. It's the best pose to start slowly letting go of anxiety and stress. Allow the breath to flow naturally. You don't need to control it here as you ease into the beginning of your practice.

Relax in your Child's Pose for a couple of minutes breathing gently.

For this, bring the big toes to touch, the knees may be wide or close together. Inhale to get ready. Exhale; lower your hips to your heels and place your belly between your thighs. Place the arms on the mat. Choose to move the arms down the sides of the legs for a more restorative impact. Breathe deeply in the pose for 1-4 minutes.

Stay relaxed, calm, and breathe. Press gently on your hands and knees and get on your back. Stay still for a moment before you proceed.

Setu Bandhasana (Bridge Pose)

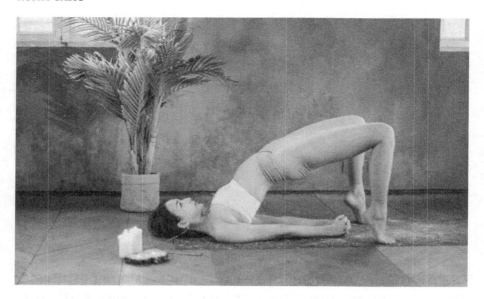

Bringing your head below the level of your heart is calming in nature, and the Bridge Pose is a perfect one to start with. This pose is a great "Timeout" from heat. You may perform this at midday, evening, or any moment you need to cool down!

There's a reason we tend to do Bridge Pose towards the end of the practice. It's a cooling down posture—the perfect way to bring the heated Pitta back into balance. Just like you did in your Cat/Cow, feel that belly fire spread to your pelvis, hips, legs, and legs. This version of it is a Pitta pleaser. You may also do this by using a block under the sacrum or unsupported.

Perform Bridge Pose as you normally should (feet apart from the hip-width, feel through the entire surface of the sole of your feet), but keep your shoulders level to the floor. Bend the elbows and lightly press the triceps down to the floor.

Broaden across the collarbones, slightly lifting the chin. Engage your belly (navel in and up) and soften your glutes a little, but not so much that you feel it in your lower back. Focus on cooling, calming, and relaxing here for 4-6 breaths, and then bring your hip down slowly. Repeat 3 times.

Savasana (Corpse Pose)

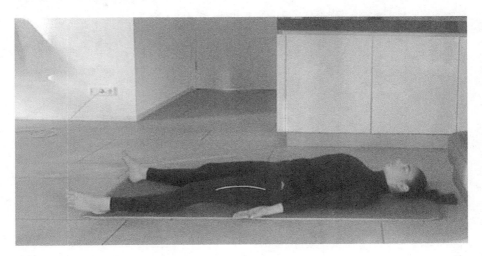

Lie on the mat. Extend the legs straight with the legs as wide as the mat. Place the left hand over the space of the heart and the right hand over the belly. Scan your body from head to foot, observe the relaxing and calming results of your Pitta balancing practice.

See how, by resting your left hand on your heart, you automatically draw your breath and attention to that region. Focus on a feeling of gratitude. One thing you can be grateful for is the deep love and happiness. Take a deep, audible breath through your mouth and exhale. Soften every muscle; release any holding or physical tension. Relax the mind, still the thoughts.

Close the eyes and surrender to the cool darkness of the eyelids as you integrate the body into silence and stillness. Rest in Savasana for 5-10 minutes.

Kaki Pranayama (Beak Breath)

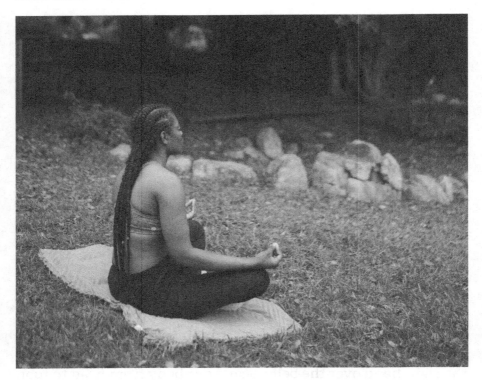

Beak Breath is a yogic calming technique that pacifies the Pitta Dosha. It elongates the inhalation and reduces the speed of breathing, which tends to minimize Pitta imbalances— anger, dissatisfaction, and tension. This breathing technique is performed by pulsing the lips to create a slight "O" shape on the inhalation, producing a feeling close to that of drinking through the straw.

At the top of the inhalation, the mouth closes and the exhalation is through the nose. The inhalation through the mouth gives a cooling feeling to the tongue that helps dispel the heat from the body.

When you're ready, sit in your comfortable position. If required, maybe place a pillow under the bones to support the spine. Close your eyes and begin the practice of Kaki Breath. Include 2-3 beat holding (breathing) before each exhalation. Practice this pranayama for around 3-5 minutes, holding your breath as gentle as possible.

Padma Mudra (Lotus Pose)

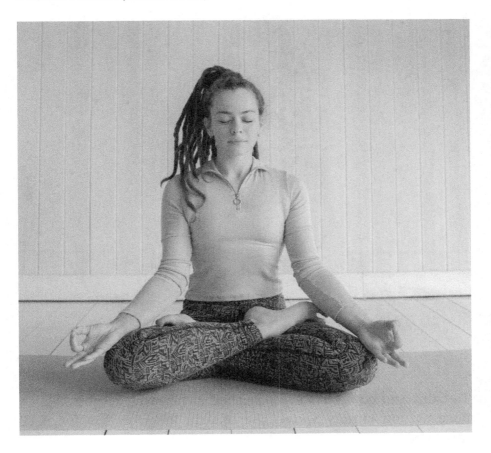

Sit and fold your legs in the way shown in the picture. Let your hand rest on your leg with your index finger and thumb joined. Keep your spine straight and chest open.

Close your eyes and encourage caring thoughts of love and appreciation to invade your mind. Padma or Lotus Mudra calms the body and mind, supports digestion issues, and binds the Heart Chakra, welcoming the energy of compassion and forgiveness that can help stabilize the Pitta Dosha.

Seated Meditation

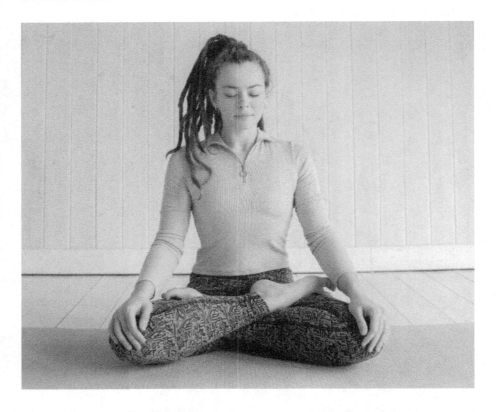

To calm and cool Pitta even further, ease into the cross-legged pose as you simply watch the breath. Practice this for 5-10 minutes.

Some Other Poses

Dhanurasana (Bow Pose) is also an excellent Solar Plexus extension pose for Pitta. It may play a role in the treatment of ulcers and hepatitis, too.

From Experience

• It is important for individuals with Pitta Dosha to avoid extremes. Gentle yoga is good for the Pitta type to blow off steam. Like if you do Namaskars, begin with Chandra Namaskar (Moon Salutation) rather than Surya Namaskar (Sun Salutation). Chandra Namaskar is much more gentle, calming, and nurturing. Visualize the navel and Solar Plexus regions getting rejuvenated when doing it.

• Just because a session has an overall cooling effect does not mean it can't also be challenging. Classes can, for example, focus on creating a steady, strong foundation or on uplifting backbends, while at the same time providing a substantial physical and/or mental challenge—all without being too heating. It's all in how you approach the practice.

PITTA BALANCING HERBS

From the Ayurvedic point of view, the mind naturally is calm and clear. Pitta Dosha may disturb this calmness and increase heat in the body. You need to use a variety of lifestyle steps like diet, meditation, yoga, and seasonal guidelines to manage the dosha. But Ayurvedic herbs provide an additional edge not only to maintain balance but also to treat dosha imbalances as and when they occur.

Ayurveda recommends taking certain herbs that are suited to the body's needs; these special herbs are very helpful in bringing the aggravated Pitta back to balance.

This part of the book contains several herbs from the Indian subcontinent that have been used and applied in Ayurveda for thousands of years. Below is the list of herbs you need to balance your Pitta Dosha:

Shatavari (Asparagus racemosus)

• It is a Vata and Pitta rejuvenative that promotes vitality and strength.

• It is a nourishing tonic for men and women.

• It maintains a healthy reproductive system for women.

• It promotes healthy lactation.

• It promotes fertility and healthy libido.

• It strengthens and rejuvenates tissues.

• It moisturizes and softens the skin.

• It supports gentle detoxification.

• It supports breast health.

• Taste: Bitter

• Energetics: Cooling

Botanically referred to as Asparagus racemosus, Shatavari is a typical Ayurvedic stimulant that is capable of rejuvenating the body. Ayurvedic literature classifies it as one of the most essential herbs or Rasayanas used to promote strength and longevity.

Studies suggest that the herb enhances the immune response by improving the activity of macrophages—the immune cells responsible for digesting highly harmful pathogens and cancer cells.

Scientists have also observed that Shatavari helps the immune system heal more rapidly from exposure to contaminants by shielding blood-producing cells in the bone marrow and by stimulating the development of immune-regulating messenger molecules.

Shatavari is a sweet and bitter herb with soothing, heavy, and oily effects, making it the best fit for pacifying the aggravated Pitta. In fact, it comes with a nourishing, calming impact that the Pitta constitution individuals will benefit from.

Thanks to the combination of these properties, Shatavari has been widely used to encourage good reproductive and digestive safety, as well as blood purity and flow. As one study suggested, Shatavari is a galactagogue plant that shows a substantial capacity for enhanced lactation.

Shatavari, native to India, belongs to the same family as the common asparagus and has nourishing, calming, and relaxing properties that aid with several situations under which the body and mind are overheated, tired, or out of control. Such symptoms can involve heartburn, indigestion, diarrhea, urinary tract infection, and irritable bowel syndrome.

It is also widely used for disorders impacting the female reproductive system, including mood swings and irritation associated with premenstrual syndrome, as well as menopausal hot flashes. Often interpreted as "She who possesses 100 husbands," Shatavari also has a reputation as a fertility-enhancing plant that enhances the well-being of both male and female reproductive tissues. It is often recommended to increase the quality of breast milk in nursing mothers, although there has been relatively little scientific research to verify its efficacy in this field.

The prescribed dosage is 500-1,000 mg twice daily.

Brahmi (Bacopa monnieri)

• It's an anti-inflammatory herb used in the treatment of anemia and chronic fever.

• It is used in the treatment of skin diseases, inflammation, and itching.

• It is used in the treatment of spleen disorders.

• It improves health, quality of life, and acts as an anti-aging medication.

• It is claimed to boost attention, intellect, and memory and to be effective in the treatment of psychiatric disorders.

• It is used in the treatment of speech impairment problems.

• It functions as a heart tonic that controls blood flow. • It's anti-diabetic effects help to reduce and stabilize blood sugar levels.

• Its anti-diabetic effects help to reduce and stabilize blood sugar levels.

• It is used to treat asthma, chronic bronchial problems, cough, and cold.

• Taste: Bitter, sweet

• Energetics: Cooling

Brahmi is a rejuvenating herb in the botanical medicine chest of Ayurveda. It has a calming effect on our physiology and has been traditionally used to help the optimum functioning of the nervous system and improve memory, learning, and focus.

This adaptogenic herb is so highly revered in Ayurvedic medicine that it has crowned the name Brahmi, a derivation of the term Brahman, which means "The energy of universal consciousness." (Gotu Kola and other natural herbs are also often referred to as Brahmi, so be sure to read the list of ingredients while purchasing it).

Unsurprisingly, Brahmi holds the position of supremacy and divinity in both the Hindu religion and the Ayurvedic culture. It is an essential component in several traditional Ayurvedic medicines and is now commonly used in herbal therapies.

The herb can treat venereal infections, nervous disorders, senility, epilepsy, hair loss, inflammatory skin problems, and premature aging. As characterized by its bitter and astringent taste and sweet post-digestive effect, Brahmi makes an excellent tridoshic remedy that is particularly soothing to Pitta.

As recent experiments have also demonstrated, Brahmi has a profound impact on the nervous system and has an enormous ability to improve memory and mental well-being. Brahmi oil massages are considered to provide a calming impact on the mind and can also be used to facilitate relaxation and sleep.

The prescribed dosage depends on the overall amount of the

Bacoside (active compound) in the formulation, although it is usually safe to take 1-3 grams a day.

Triphala (Three Fruits)

• It's a balancing formula for detoxification and rejuvenation.

• It supports natural internal cleaning.

• It gently maintains regularity.

• It nourishes and rejuvenates tissues.

• It supports healthy digestion and absorption.

• It is a natural antioxidant.

• Tastes: Sweet, sour, pungent, bitter, astringent

• Energetic: Neutral (heating and cooling)

Triphala is an herbal blend made from the fruit of 3 trees growing in India and the Middle East (the Sanskrit term Triphala means "Three Fruits"). The 3 fruits are Amalaki (Emblica officinalis), Bibhitaki (Terminalia bellirica), and Haritaki (Terminalia chebula). Amalaki is cooling, while Bibhitaki and Haritaki are hot.

Amalaki (Emblica officinalis), commonly referred to as Indian gooseberry or Amla, is considered to be one of the best rejuvenating herbs in Ayurveda. Traditionally, it has been used to combat skin diseases, respiratory disorders, diabetes, asthma, and indigestion. Amalaki is a strong natural antioxidant with high levels of vitamin C. In India, Amalaki is known as the "Nurse Herb" because it strengthens the immune system and cools the body, balancing the Pitta Dosha.

Haritaki (Terminalia chebula) has the most laxative capacity of the three fruits found in the Triphala. In Tibet, Haritaki is so highly revered that it is often portrayed in Tibetan religious paintings in the stretched palm of the Medicine Buddha. The herb also has astringent properties and balances Vata.

Bibhitaki (Terminalia bellerica) is an excellent rejuvenator, both laxative and astringent. It eliminates excess mucus in the body, balancing the Kapha Dosha. In addition, Bibhitaki is a powerful treatment for a variety of lung conditions, including bronchitis and asthma.

The fruits are dried, ground into powder, and mixed in a precise manner established by the ancient herbalists. This balances the Vata Dosha as well as the Pitta and the Kapha. It also contains 5 of the 6 tastes, with no salty taste. The plant that makes up Triphala has powerful soothing and purifying powers.

Triphala is a particularly useful herbal blend because it gently cleanses and detoxifies the body without irritating the colon. In addition, unlike other laxatives that deplete the body, Triphala actually strengthens and nourishes the bones, nervous system, and reproductive organs.

Triphala is prescribed and is used more than any other Ayurvedic herbal formulation. Popular for its unique ability to softly disinfect and detoxify the body while continuously replenishing and nourishing it, this conventional procedure facilitates the proper functioning of the digestive, circulatory, respiratory, and genitourinary processes.

It is usually used as a daily supplement to help maintain the balance of the doshas. The recommended dose is 500-1,000 mg twice daily.

Bhringraj (Eclipta prostrata)

- It provides tranquility to mind and body.

- It supports healthy hair growth.

- It promotes natural hair color and helps with balding.

- It's a cooling rejuvenation to soothe excess Pitta.

- It supports a calm mind, healthy skin, and a radiant complexion.

- Tastes: Pungent, bitter

- Energetics: Cooling

Also known as false daisy, Bhringraj is a common medicinal herb that thrives in tropical conditions with high humidity rates. In India, the leaves of the plant are highly valued for oil that serves as a natural hair tonic and is used in many Ayurvedic hair products.

In Ayurveda, Bhringraj is known to be a tridoshic herb capable of controlling Vata, Kapha, and Pitta. The herb is especially useful in treating the worsening of Pitta and its complications, such as swelling, inflammation, and loss of hair. Nevertheless, one should ensure that the herb is used in moderation and combined with cooling herbs—mint—to prevent its heating capacity from having adverse effects on Pitta Dosha.

In addition, several studies have investigated the efficacy of Bhringraj as hair rejuvenation and found that it has the potential to be an efficient booster of hair growth.

The dosage is as follows:

- Bhringraj Juice - 1-2 teaspoons twice a day.

- Bhringraj Powder - ¼- ½ teaspoon twice a day.

- Bhringraj Capsule - 1-2 capsules twice a day.

• Bhringraj Tablet - 1-2 tablets twice a day.

Guduchi (Tinospora cordifolia)

• It increases longevity.

• It relieves burning pain.

• It relieves excess hunger.

• It improves breast milk.

• It relieves anorexia that makes a person feel hungry.

• It works as a rejuvenator.

• It has a propensity to consume the liquid content of Malas (gastric waste) giving a regular consistency.

• It increases energy.

• It inflames the digestive fire.

• It relieves the indications of aging.

• It increases control, power, memory, and recollection ability.

• Taste: Bitter, astringent

• Energetics: Heating

Guduchi or Gaduchi, medically known as Tinospora cordifolia, is now one of the most common Ayurvedic herbs to be studied for their therapeutic value. Traditionally, Guduchi has been used to combat a broad variety of diseases. The herb is generally referred to in India as 'Amrit,' the Sanskrit term for 'Immortality.'

Ayurveda sees Guduchi as an important nerve tonic that can improve the nervous system and pacify Pitta Dosha. When it is paired with a bitter and astringent taste and a sweet post-digestive effect, the herb makes an excellent remedy for soothing the irritated Pitta. It may also help to keep Vata and Kapha Dosha in check if used daily.

Although Guduchi has also been prescribed for improving immune function and purported anti-allergic properties, several studies suggest that it has a cleansing and detoxifying impact on the body. Thus, it can be used as an antioxidant source and as a medicine to cure and prevent a broad range of medical conditions.

½-1 tablespoon of Guduchi (Tinospora cordifolia) can be consumed with plain water after meals, 2 times a day.

Mint (Mentha)

• It's high in nutrients.

• It improves Irritable Bowel Syndrome. (It is a common disorder of the digestive tract.)

• It helps relieve indigestion.

• It boosts neural activity.

• It can decrease breastfeeding pain.

• It subjectively improves cold symptoms.

• It can mask bad breath.

• It's versatile enough to be added to most dishes.

• Tastes: Sweet, lingering

• Energetics: Cooling

Mint is a herb we're all familiar with. Identified as Pudina across the Indian subcontinent, it has long kept and significant role in Ayurveda and is a popular ingredient in several traditional Ayurvedic formulations and home remedies.

Although mint is available in a variety of types, including peppermint, spearmint, and horsemint, all of them are known to have tridoshic properties and may be especially beneficial in pacifying Pitta. These herbs have a sweet taste and are most notable for their soothing properties, which may help to soothe intense inner heat and its symptoms.

In addition to suppressing irritated Pitta, research also shows that mint can be used to boost digestion, boost respiratory function, and have general health benefits as an antioxidant and antiseptic agent.

Dosage is up to 1,200 mg maximum (180-400 mg 3 times daily).

Choosing Other Herbs

Although the herbs listed above have a stabilizing impact and will help hold Pitta levels in control, there are several other herbs that you can use to find the balance.

We have several insights from classical texts to understand the classification of herbs based on the Prakriti or dosha type. They prescribe herbs dependent on different tastes owing to the subsequent impact on each dosha.

Because Pitta is renowned for its hotness, sharpness, and lightness, you should avoid herbs that accentuate Pitta's heat quality. This will include herbs with pungent, sour, and salty tastes. Instead, look for sweet, bitter, and astringent herbs that can help to balance Pitta by introducing its contradictory qualities.

If you were to obey these guidelines, some more herbs that are appropriate for your dosha would include coriander, cardamom, cilantro, fennel, cumin, and turmeric.

OIL MASSAGE EFFE(
IN PITTA BALANC..

O nce we hear that word, many of us envision a luxurious spa experience reserved for special occasions. In Ayurveda, however, Abhyanga (Ayurvedic oil massage) is prescribed every day. Fortunately, there is a more affordable option to professional massage therapy when it comes to experiencing the nourishing advantages of Abhyanga every day.

But how can a routine that is so luxuriously soothing, so blissfully calming, restore the body and mind and set us up for peak performance?

There is a reason for the apparent contradiction. Accumulated pain and contaminants are eliminated from the mind and body through routine massage. A daily full-body warm oil massage, therefore, acts as a powerful recharger and rejuvenator of mind and body.

Oil massage may sound like a messy and complicated procedure that's best left to the spa, but once you've mastered the fundamentals, it becomes our second nature and worth the effort. In this section, we're going to discuss the advantages of Abhyanga, which oil to use, and how you can adapt your self-massage practice to balance Pitta Dosha.

What is Self-Massage/Abhyanga?

Self-massage, as its name suggests, is the act of massaging

elf. Ayurveda suggests gently massaging the whole body th warm oil every morning—a real treat that you wouldn't want to skip! It is an essential part of the daily regimen prescribed by this healing system for general health and well-being.

It is important to note, though, that doing Abhyanga on your own is a more involved process than just slathering some oil on your neck or back for a few minutes. It recommends spending a minimum of 15 minutes on self-massage each time you practice it, devoting love and attention to each of the tissue layers as you nourish them with warm Ayurvedic oil.

Abhyanga is a Sanskrit word, which means "Oil Massage." Also known as Abiyangam, it is a type of Ayurvedic therapy that includes a therapeutic massage of Ayurvedic oils. Unlike traditional massage therapy, Abhyanga is seen as an act of self-love and helps to promote the physical, mental, and psychological well-being of the individual.

Traditional Ayurvedic scriptures are eloquent about the advantages. Here's what one says—

"Give yourself a full-body oil massage daily. It's nourishing; pacifies the doshas; relieves fatigue; offers strength, relaxation, and great sleep; improves the skin's beauty and glow; encourages longevity; nourishes all parts of the body."

Abhyanga provides a means of transdermal absorption of the healing properties of the substance used in the massage and lets the skin—the body's largest organ—conduct its various functions effectively, whether allowing toxins to be released from the body or nourishment to be consumed by the tissues.

It's like oiling your car's engine—if you do it daily, your engine will be in top condition, bringing you years and years of trouble-free performance.

134

How do Abhyanga Works?

According to Ayurvedic scriptures, Abhyanga calms and balances the doshas in the case of abundance. Quite often we witness Pitta excess during the summer season, or we find it among Pitta type and highly stressed individuals who have difficulty falling asleep and are suffering from anxiety.

Abhyanga needs you to massage yourself thoroughly every day for at least 15 minutes so that the oil penetrates deep into your skin.

By doing so, you imitate the experience of a loving embrace and offer yourself the self-care you deserve. While the thought of an oil massage may seem complicated and challenging to do on your own, with some learning you may enjoy the full benefits of an oil massage in the comfort of your home and have a self-care routine you can enjoy each day.

Benefits of Abhyanga

Abhyanga is more than just a body massage—it's a way for you to show self-love. By offering yourself a calming oil massage, you're loving and praising yourself for being who you are. The effects of Abhyanga are physical, emotional, and intellectual, and can help people of all ages and all walks of life.

As long as you choose the right massage oil for yourself and take care of your towels and clothing, a regular massage can be a basic and extremely special part of your routine.

So, enable yourself to enjoy your "Me-time" and set aside time each day for an Ayurvedic oil massage—you will experience long-term benefits and a heightened sense of well-being and happiness amidst the chaos of daily life.

Although it is often advised to seek massage from a skilled massage therapist, there is much to be gained from practicing and using Ayurvedic self-massage techniques. By performing self-massage, the wonderful advantages of Abhyanga will be readily available to you in the comfort of your own home. It, over time, becomes a daily act of self-love that you can look forward to every day.

In fact, the benefits of Abhyanga go beyond stress relief. Massage in Ayurveda is prescribed as an outstanding treatment that can enhance the functioning of the nervous system, restore sleep cycles, promote healthy hair and skin, strengthen the limbs, and improve overall lifespan.

Massage is also a good way to lose extra body weight because oils act as fat burners when thoroughly massaged into the skin. If you suffer from dry or barren skin, Abhyanga can contribute to a noticeable improvement in the quality of your skin as the oils function to restore the tissues and reverse the effects of dehydration, aging, and wrinkles.

Plus, the soothing powers of Abhyanga oils extract toxins from the body and improve the overall function of the internal organs.

Over time, a daily Abhyanga routine promotes the equilibrium of Ayurvedic doshas in the body and enhances lifespan. The practice of Abhyanga is deemed an expression of self-love and nourishes the body and mind in the same way as the feeling of being deeply loved.

Here are some benefits traditionally associated with regular performance of this pleasant daily ritual:

• **Massage Helps Maintain or Restore Circulation:** Appropriate massage helps to maintain or stimulate circulation in the body. Typically, a part of the body that has become rigid or flabby has poor circulation and little sensation. Massaging these areas may help to restore adequate circulation and nervous system function.

• **Massage Provides a Purifying and Cleansing Influence:** Massage has a purifying and detoxifying effect on physiology. When we rub and squeeze our skin and body, we help break up the cumulative layers of toxins and impurities that have been trapped in the tissues and disrupt the fragile biochemistry. Massage often induces heat and friction, which improves the movement of fluids through the blood and lymph vessels. It tends to clean and open up these essential circulation pathways.

• **Massage Maintains the Suppleness and Youthfulness of the Skin:** Massage preserves the suppleness and youthfulness of the skin. When the body is massaged with warm oil, some of it is absorbed by the skin. Even after showering, the skin stays soft and supple. Oil massage helps prevent the skin from becoming dry and helps maintain its youthfulness.

• **Massage Provides a Stabilizing and Balancing Effect on Pitta:** Coconut oil is one of the healthiest of all Pitta substances. Classic symptoms of Pitta disorder include exhaustion, fatigue, excess heat, digestive problems, and distracting feeling. When the entire body surface has consumed coconut oil from massage, these effects are decreased and there is greater evenness, strength, and stability throughout the day.

• **Massage Increases the Secretion of Hormones from the Skin:** Massage increases the secretion of hormones from the skin. These hormones, such as growth hormones, endorphins, etc., help to give the body power and immunity.

Why is Massage Recommended in Ayurveda?

The practice of massage itself takes the stress and tension away from the muscles. And these effects are further strengthened by the addition of dosha-pacifying oil. Health benefits from incorporating a regular oil rub into your morning or evening routine include:

• Wellness of the musculoskeletal and nervous system

• Good circulation and lymphatic drainage

• Improved sleep habits

• Smoother, healthier skin

• Healthy vision

• Graceful aging

• Lascivious hair

• Solid, strong limbs

• Strength and vigor for body tissues

• Enhanced durability

• Nourishment for the whole body

When to Practice?

It can be practiced before a morning shower or a soothing evening bath (I prefer it in the evening since it's great for sleep). Abhyanga is a great daily practice if you have time, or at least try to get one on the weekend. It's always done before you get in the shower/bath so that the extra oil that isn't consumed can be washed away instead of rubbing all over your clothing.

It's best to use some oil after your shower or bath to keep your skin moist, but be sure you're completely dry before applying so that it's not clogging. (I prefer coconut oil.)

Why is Abhyanga a Potent Stress Reliever?

There is an explanation of why Abhyanga's oil self-massage has been an integral part of the Ayurvedic daily morning ritual for thousands of years. Massage alone is strongly recommended as a way to relax the body's muscles and relieve internal stress. Throughout Ayurveda, the beneficial effects of massage are claimed to be improved by including Ayurvedic massage oil.

The feelings of Ayurvedic massage mimic the impression of a warm embrace, calming tension and mental stress, and infusing you with peace and contentment.

The Sanskrit term "Sneha" translates to "love" as well as "oil," and Ayurveda stresses this intrinsic connection between the feeling of love and the body in oil. The feeling of "Sneha," be it love or oil, is a gentle one (Sukshma) that enables it to penetrate through the smallest channels of the body through its seven layers of tissue (Dhatus). Massage also helps improve blood circulation and thus ease tension within the body, which further decreases stress levels.

Which Oil to Choose?

Ayurveda is all about finding the right balance in the body. According to Ayurveda, the opposites balance each other out, and like enhances like. When you choose massage oil for yourself, it is therefore important to choose one that corrects the imbalances in your body.

To do this, you need to take into account the Ayurvedic doshas— Vata, Pitta, and Kapha—and how these doshas have an effect on various aspects of your life. Such things shall involve:

Vikriti – This is the current level of balance of your body. If one of the doshas in your body is currently high, it is best to choose a massage oil that will pacify the specific dosha. For example, if you happen to have anxiety and your body's temperature is low, you are likely to have high rates of Vata Dosha, so you should choose an oil that pacifies Vata.

Prakriti – This is the overall Ayurvedic structure of your body. If the doshas in your body are more or less balanced, you should take into account the prevailing dosha in your body's structure while receiving a massage oil. For example, if your dominant body is Pitta and the weather is hot and humid, your Pitta may get worse, so you should choose an oil that pacifies Pitta.

Seasons – There is a strong link between the seasons and the doshas. Summer is called a Pitta season, fall to early winter is a Vata season, and late winter to spring is a Kapha season. There are several steps you can take to preserve your body's equilibrium over different seasons, and choosing the right Ayurvedic massage oil is one of them.

For Pitta (someone who's a little more oily, sharp, heated, and emotionally distracted), you don't need a lot; coconut oil in its purest form is perfect for you.

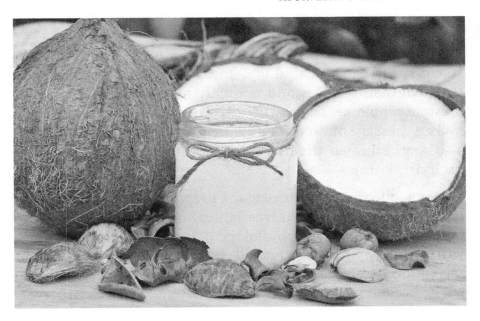

Coconut is a joy for the senses and the body, a symbol of tropical paradise. It is said, "It has a sweet and tropical taste that reminds of an island in the Caribbean by the shore." This idyllic and enjoyable tree nut restores balance and harmony.

Coconut oil is sweet, cool, and nourishing, but exceptionally light. It's the perfect liver tonic.

Research reveals that around 65% of the material you place on the skin is absorbed into the bloodstream. Ayurveda implies that you shouldn't place anything on your skin that you wouldn't eat. Thus, you can feel good when rubbing coconut oil on your skin.

Because coconut oil is soothing, it's great for self-massage during the summer months, in warm climates, or if you're somebody who's constantly hot. If you are a cold sort, use sesame oil, which is warm. If you are a cold sort, use sesame oil, which is warm. You can also blend the coconut oil with sesame oil during winter. This way, it's going to be a little cooling and little warming. (Additional benefit: The heat of the sesame oil leaves the coconut oil in the liquid state during winter.)

Alternatively, it can be used as a basis for other herbal oils. For starters, Ashwagandha oil is renowned for its effective ability to strengthen muscles and is highly recommended for active lifestyle supplements. You should combine it with coconut oil to make a massage oil solution that helps build muscle mass while also soothing. (But the use of just coconut oil is also great for pacifying Pitta).

Coconut oil contains antioxidant properties and is helpful in protecting the skin from free radical damage. It is known to be highly nutritious for physiology. The complete body massage with warm, pure coconut oil is not only an epitome of relaxation; it also stimulates the immune system and has a purifying and relaxing effect on the body and mind of Pitta type.

Just remember to buy organic oils all the time; the skin will consume them, and the body will absorb them just like water. Coconut oil can be distilled (less fragrance) or unrefined (traditional oil used), just don't seek those so-called pure coconut oil filled with preservatives and chemicals.

Thus, choose high-quality, chemical-free organic coconut oil to get the best results from your massage therapy.

So, How is the Abhyanga Done?

You'll have to do Abhyanga in your bathroom just before you take a bath. Use slightly warm massage oil. (Store the oil in a plastic flip-top and warm it by keeping the bottle under running hot water for a few minutes).

Follow the steps:

• When doing your Ayurvedic massage, it is important to be completely relaxed, so choose a day when you have enough time on your hands.

• Choose a warm, comfortable room away from the wind where you can stand or sit while you massage.

• Make sure the skin is clean and dry so that it can easily absorb hydrating oil. You should massage the skin by cleaning it with a dry brush to avoid any dirt or dead skin cells.

• Warm the oil. Check the temperature by placing a drop on your inner wrist, the oil should be comfortably warm and not hot.

• Sit or stand comfortably.

• Apply oil first to the crown of your head (Adhipati Marma; home to many other essential Marma points—points of focused vital energy) and work slowly out of it in circular strokes, spending a few minutes massaging the whole scalp.

• Face: Massage in a circular motion on your forehead, temples, cheeks, and jaws (always moving upward). Be sure to massage your ears, particularly your ear lobes—home to vital Marma points and nerve endings.

• Perform long strokes on the limbs (arms and legs) and short strokes on the joints (elbows and knees). Always massage towards the direction of your heart.

• Massage your abdomen and chest in a big, clockwise, circular motion. Follow the path of the large intestine on the abdomen; move up on the right side of the abdomen, then down on the left side of the abdomen.

• Complete the massage by spending at least a few minutes massaging your feet. Feet are a very critical part of the body with the nerve endings of the internal organs and crucial Marma points.

• Sit with oil for 5-15 minutes, if necessary, so that the oil will absorb and enter the deeper layers of the body. The longer the oil is on, the more the oil penetrates. During this time, you can read something relaxing or rest; or you can shave, trim your nails, and get ready for the day. Dab excess oil off with paper towels if you like, then follow with a soothing hot bath or shower.

• Enjoy a warm bath or shower. You can use a gentle soap on the "strategic" regions; avoid intense soaping and rubbing.

• As you get out of the water, pat yourself gently with a towel. Blot the towel on your body instead of rubbing aggressively.

• To further elevate the experience, apply some essential oils to your neck and wrists after bathing. (Use coconut oil)

Enjoy the feeling of having nourished your body, mind, and soul and carry it with you all day long. And if your schedule doesn't qualify for a regular massage, try to squeeze it at least 3-4 times a week. You'll find it worth it!

Pro Tip: To promote healthy sleep patterns, rub the scalp and soles of the legs with sesame oil before bedtime.

Oil Pulling with Coconut Oil (A Complete Body Detox within 20 Minutes)

If you know anything about oil pulling you know how helpful it can be, and with the oil that favors your body type, it'll take your health and fitness game to the next level.

As you may know that our tongue is linked to various important parts of the body, that's why your doctor often tells you to show your tongue when they examine you.

Doing oil pulling eliminates all the toxins from your body no matter how long they have been in existence. Oil pulling does so because in our body contaminants are found in the form of oils, so when you do oil pulling, it absorbs the toxins and you get a full detox within 15-20 minutes.

To use sesame oil as part of your daily oral regimen, take one tablespoon of oil in the morning and swish in the mouth. Don't gargle and don't swallow. Swish for up to 20 minutes (you may need to build up to this), allowing the oil and the saliva to form a yellowish mixture in your mouth. Spit and clean the mouth with warm water. You may follow a rinse with a mouthwash or brush your teeth to remove any leftover residue.

Post Massage Cleaning

As you might have expected, Abhyanga will leave a mess in the bathroom. It can leave splotches of oil on the walls, the floors, and the tub. So to ensure that your space stays clean and laundry is minimally impaired, keep a separate towel to sit on during your massage and a separate towel to dry after your shower.

In addition, if you are doing Abhyanga at night, wear a separate set of cotton nightclothes after your shower for at least an hour before sleeping to remove some excess oil. You can also place a towel around your mattress before you sleep so that any remaining oil in your hair is absorbed.

During your shower, you should wash the bathtub quickly with a lot of dish soap. This will save it from building up and you're going to love having a warm bath every time you shower!

Besides, you're never going to have to scour it again with chemicals, because the dish soap can hold it extra clean. It only takes a minute to wash it out since you do it every time. I also noticed that this mixed solution is effective in preventing the build-up of oily clogs in the pipes.

Another convenient way to protect your clothing is by adding a distilled combination of vinegar and soda to the washing machine while washing clothes. Though corrosive in large quantities, this is excellent for eliminating oil stains when mixed with hot water. You can also use a natural, environment-friendly detergent to wash your clothes.

One last thing to remember is that oil is highly flammable, so be cautious when drying oily towels and clothing. Ideally, you should let them dry naturally, but if you use a cloth dryer, use at a low-heat setting so that they are not at risk of catching fire. You should also be careful not to leave oil-stained clothes or towels in your bathroom.

Coconut Oil and Ayurveda: Traditional Uses

According to Ayurveda, coconut oil has Pitta and Vata pacifying properties. It nourishes and strengthens immunity and strength. Coconut oil includes rare Medium-Chain Fatty Acids (MCFAs) that are quickly and readily ingested, digested, metabolized, and used by the body. They don't clog arteries like longer-chained fats or spike blood sugar.

It has a high smoking point, and it does not cause cancer-causing free radicals when used for cooking. It is known to be the best massage oil for newborns and infants. It soothes the baby's diaper rash and dry skin.

Coconut oil self-massage is highly recommended for these benefits:

• It's a perfect coolant.

• Its digestion requires a fairly long period.

• Improves the quality and strength of the hair.

• Promotes the growth of hair.

• It's a natural aphrodisiac.

• Protects the delicate lining of the small and large intestine.

• Promotes cardiac protection when consumed with a whole-food, plant-based diet.

• Supports a healthy immune system as it is antibacterial, antifungal, and antiviral.

• Helps control metabolism.

• Provides stamina and vitality.

• Ideal for memory and brain functioning.

• Decreases inflammation, including gum inflammation and arthritis-related inflammation.

• Moisturizes the skin when used both internally and externally.

• It also accelerates the healing process of the wound in the body.

• Nourishes undernourished body tissues.

• Effective in the diagnosis of other illnesses such as emaciation, fatigue, respiratory problems, diabetes, and urinary system problems.

• Quickens and helps in filling up skin depression in wounds.

• Calms Vata, Pitta, and supports Kapha.

Contraindications

Coconut oil should be avoided from an Ayurvedic viewpoint if there is excess cooling in the body as well as excessive Ama (toxic build-up) or inflammation.

Oil Massage: Practical Hacks

1.Overall, oil massage usually takes 10-15 minutes but can be done in only around 5 minutes by reducing the number of strokes in each spot. (Only for those lazy days.)

2. Apply the oil to all parts of your body before you start the massage stroke. This will cause the oil to be in your body for a longer amount of time before you take a bath or shower.

3. Ideally, leave the oil on for up to 20 minutes after the massage before taking a bath or a shower. But, if the time does not allow you to leave the oil on, you can bathe or shower directly afterward.

4. If you don't wash your hair daily, you may have an oil massage each day on all parts of your body other than your head. Massage your head with oil on the days you want to wash your hair.

5. It can also be performed in the evening if the morning is not appropriate for you.

Some Common FAQs about Oil Massages

What is the Significance of Oils?

Carefully extracted from plants,highly nutritious oils have been coveted over the centuries. Anointing with oil has a long history throughout the globe, as far back as ancient Egyptian days when oil was believed to have both spiritual and physical effects and used to recognize someone as a leader—whether a Pharaoh or a husband.
The practice is present in many other cultures and regions, including Greek mythology, aboriginal Australia. Some East African groups, as well as Buddhism, Hinduism, and Christianity promotes it. In many of these civilizations, anointing was believed to have healing properties, including Ayurveda. In many of these civilizations, anointing was believed to have healing properties, including Ayurveda.

Do I Have to Perform Abhyanga Myself?

Although performing self-massage is much easier than you think and is a more convenient and affordable way of treating yourself to Abhyanga (or Udvartana) regularly, you can also seek professional massage at an Ayurvedic spa. But I highly recommend you do it in your home; you'll find it easier to opt this into your routine, plus it hardly takes over 20 minutes.

What are the Benefits of Applying Oil to Hair? (Murdha Taila)

· It makes hair grow lavishly, thick, gentle, and effortless.

· It relieves and strengthens the sense organs.

· It removes facial wrinkles.

What are the Benefits of Applying Oil to Ears? (Karna Puran)

· Ear disorders due to enhanced Pitta get balanced.

· It betters neck stiffness.

· It helps in making jaws stronger.

What are the Benefits of Applying Oil to Feet? (Padaghata)

· Lightness, stiffness, roughness, fatigue, and numbness of the limbs are reduced.

· Stability and firmness of the legs are achieved.

· Sight is improved.

- Pitta is pacified.

- Sciatica decreases.

- Improves regional muscles and ligaments.

SOME PITTA PACIFYING RECIPES

Chilled Avocado and Mango Salsa

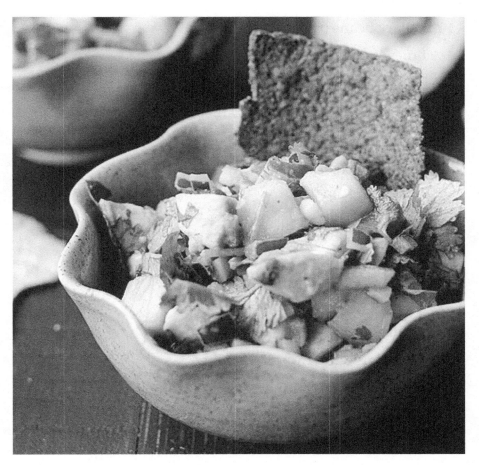

Buttery avocado and cold sweet mango in this filling dish provide healthy monounsaturated fat, fiber, and a strong dose of vitamin C. Fiber improves digestive processes, while vitamin C leads to the formation of collagen fibers (which play a crucial role in the integrity of the skin, muscles, and intestinal integrity). As an antioxidant, vitamin C also stimulates the immune system functions and decreases inflammation in the body.

Servings: 3

Ingredients:

- 1 can black beans (rinsed and drained)
- 1 ½ limes (juiced)
- ½ cup fresh cilantro (chopped)
- 1 can sweet corn (rinsed and drained)
- 2 avocados (peeled, pitted, and diced)
- 3 mangoes (peeled, pitted, and diced)
- 1 red onion (diced)
- 2 tsp extra virgin olive oil
- ½ tsp chilli powder
- Salt and pepper to taste

Instructions:

1. Within a large pot, mix all ingredients.

2. Cover and chill for a minimum of 30 minutes.

3. Eat with baked vegetables or corn chips, raw or grilled vegetables, or even spoonful... The options are infinite!

Coconut Truffles

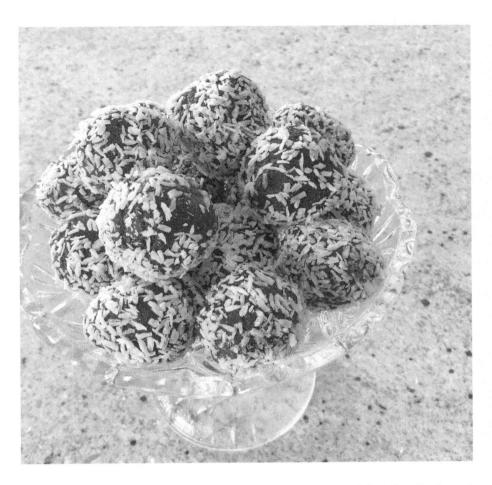

Feeling thirsty or constipated? Coconut is a friend of Pittas! These coconut truffles regulate the acid levels and cool the digestive tract.

Servings: 3

Ingredients:

- 4 cups shredded coconut

- 1 cup honey

- 2 ginger

- 1 cup dark chocolate chips

- 3 cardamom

- 4-5 saffron threads

Instructions:

1. Grind the threads of saffron, cardamom, and ginger. Melt some dark chocolate in the pan. (Pro tip: It's better to have dark chocolate chips containing cocoa.)

2. Add the sliced coconut and honey to the ground mixture to make a dough.

3. Coin out small ball-like bits or you may use any funky patterns to offer shape to your taste.

4. Cover up the baking tray with parchment paper. Dip the bits in the melting chocolate and place them on the tray.

5. You can add a little garnish by sprinkling some coconut sugar. Freeze the truffles for one hour and they'll be ready to serve.

Khichdi (Rice and Lentils Mix)

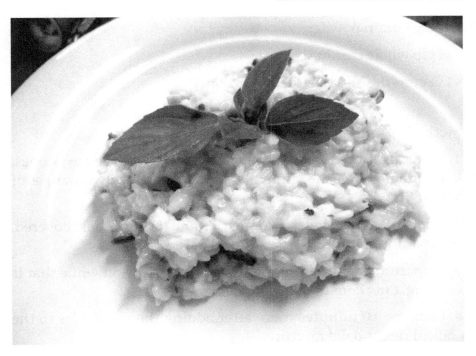

Servings: 2

Ingredients:

- ½ cup basmati rice
- 1 cup mung dal
- 6 cups water
- 2 tsp ghee
- 1-inch ginger root (chopped or grated)
- ½ tsp mustard seeds
- A handful of fresh cilantro leaves
- ½ tsp coriander powder
- ½ tsp turmeric powder
- ¼ tsp or so salt
- 1 pinch hing

- ½ tsp cumin powder
- ½ tsp whole cumin seeds
- 1½ cups desired vegetables (optional)

Method:

1. Select over the rice and dal cautiously to remove any stones. Each should be washed individually with at least two changes of water.

2. Add the 6 cups of water to the rice and dal and cook, covered, for 20 minutes, or until the rice and dal are soft.

3. Prepare any vegetables that fit your constitution while that is cooking. Cut them into bite-sized bits.

4. Cook for 10 minutes more after adding the vegetables to the cooked rice and dal mixture.

5. In a separate saucepan, sauté the seeds in ghee before they pop. Then add the remaining spices.

6. Add all the ingredients and mix thoroughly to release flavors. Mix the cooked dal, rice, and vegetable mixture with the sautéed spices.

7. Garnish with salt and fresh cilantro, if used, and serve.

Suggestions:

1. Khichdi, made with old rice and split mung dal, is good for fever or stomach ailments.

2. It is best to consume with ghee or butter throughout breastfeeding.

3. You can make a variation with basmati rice if you have weak digestive power.

4. Red rice consists of iron and zinc in the husk. Black and purple rice contain high levels of protein, fat, and essential fiber. They are helpful in tissue fatigue induced by Vata imbalance. So, make sure you include these nourishing and building foods in your recipes.

Milk and Rice Kheer (Split Rice Pudding)

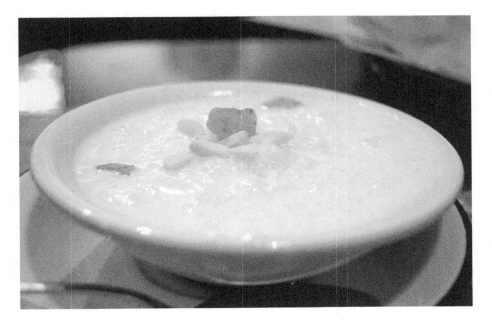

Servings: 1

Ingredients:

- 4 cups of milk (or coconut milk if vegan)

- 1 tsp ghee or vegan butter

- ½ cup of raw red rice

- 1 tsp cashew nuts

- 1 tsp raisins

- 3 green cardamoms
- 1 tsp brown or candy sugar

Instructions:

1. Soak the split red rice in water for 2 hours. Add the rice (drained of the water) into the milk and boil it.   Add the sugar once the mixture thickens.

2. Sauté the cashews in the ghee until they turn golden brown in another pan.

3. Add the raisins and cardamom and sauté.

4. Add this to the thick mixture. Serve hot.

Cucumber Raita

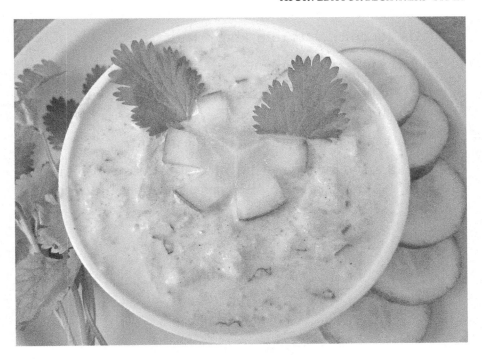

What's going to be more fun than chomping on a tasty cucumber Raita with an Indian twist! Yogurt is renowned for its soothing properties and it will provide the body with the necessary hydration.

Servings: 2

Ingredients:

- 1 cucumber

- 2 cups of yogurt

- 2 tsp cumin seeds

- 1 tsp mustard seeds

- Salt to taste

Instructions:

1. Cut the cucumber into thin, long pieces.

2. Crush the mustard seeds and the cumin seeds in the grinder.

3. Add the sliced cucumber to the yogurt. Keep the cucumber in the yogurt for 2 minutes.

4. Add the crushed spices and salt to the mixture.

5. If you like, top it with ice and allow it to cool for the next 10 minutes. You can garnish it with leaves of peppermint.

Sesame Seed Bars

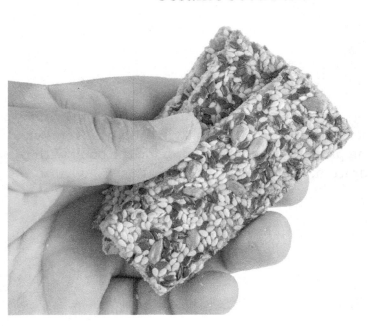

A snack made of healthy fats including seeds, nuts, and ghee.

Servings: 8

Ingredients:

- 1 cup coconut
- ¼ cup melted ghee or vegan butter
- 1 cup maple syrup
- 4 dates (chopped well)
- 4 cup sesame seeds
- 1 tsp vanilla
- ½ cup sunflower seeds
- ¾ cup cashews (well chopped)
- Sea salt to taste

Instructions:

1. Mix all the ingredients together well.

2. Oil the parchment paper and press the mix onto the paper

3. Bake in a preheated 350° oven for 10-15 minutes.

4. Cool, then cut or break into pieces.

Okra Sabzi (A Tridoshic Recipe)

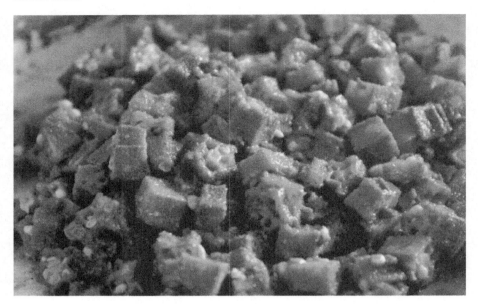

Okra is soft and slender and provides a Pitta calming impact being a coolant. It has stress and dryness relieving qualities which makes it perfect for joints, reproductive tissue, constipation, and overall healthy strength (thus, it's Vata balancing as well). It's easy to digest when cooked.

Servings: 2

Ingredients:

• ½ green chilli (chopped)

• 1-pound fresh okra (can be found at Indian and Asian grocery stores)

• 1 tsp sunflower oil or ghee

• 1 tsp cumin seeds

• 1 tsp black mustard seeds

• ½ tsp salt

Instructions:

1. Wash and dry the okra, then trim the tops and bottoms. Cut into ¼" rings.

2. Heat oil or ghee in a saucepan over medium heat. Add the seeds of cumin and mustard. After they pop, add the chilli and salt, stir until brown.

3. Add the okra, cover, and cook for around 15 minutes until tender. Stir frequently to prevent burning.

4. Serve with roti or rice.

Some Healthy Drinks

Pitta Tea

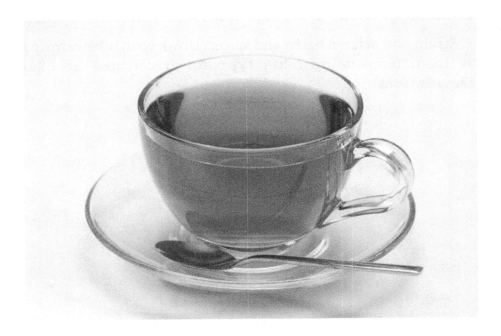

Servings: 1

Ingredients:

- 1 cup boiling water
- ¼ tsp fennel
- ¼ tsp fresh cilantro
- ¼ tsp cumin seeds
- ¼ tsp coriander
- ¼ tsp rose petals

Instructions:

1. Mix together the cumin seeds, coriander, fennel, cilantro, and rose petals.

2. Add the hot water to it. Steep for the next 5 minutes, covered.

3. Strain and discard herbs and spices. Drink cool, lukewarm, or at room temperature (Pitta type are exacerbated by high temperatures).

Golden Milk

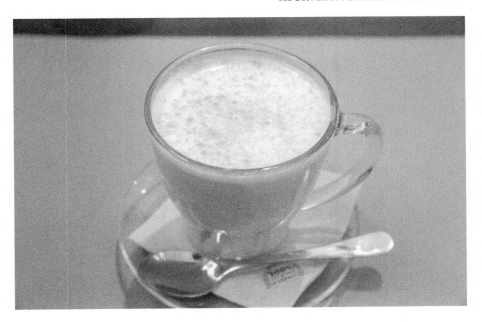

Servings: 2

Ingredients:

• 2 cups of fresh milk

• 2 tsp turmeric powder (or a 2-inch coin
of fresh turmeric root, peeled)

• A dusting of fresh cracked pepper (or a small
pinch of ground cardamom, or both)

Instructions:

1. Add the ingredients in the saucepan.

2. Gently whisk the milk and put it to a gentle simmer.

3. Serve and enjoy slightly warm.

Ayurveda Energy Drink

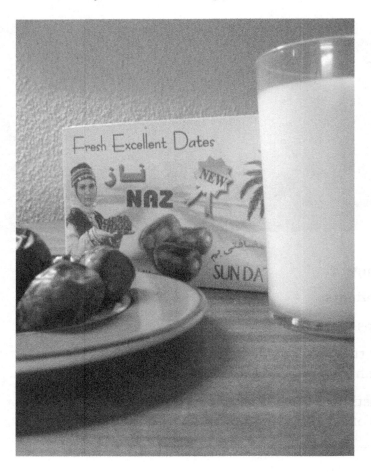

Servings: 2

Ingredients:

- 10 whole almonds (soaked overnight with skins removed)
- 2 cups of cow's milk or unsweetened almond milk
- 2 whole Medjool fresh dates (soaked overnight)

- 1 tsp ghee (or vegan butter)
- 1 pinch of cardamom powder
- 1 pinch of saffron

Instructions:

1. Place the prepared almonds in a blender with ½ cup of milk (add the milk of your choice) and mix until smooth.

3. Add the remaining ingredients and blend until smooth. Enjoy!

The trick to calming the Pitta during the summer is to ground, nourish, and stay cool. Keep Pitta balanced with these grounding recipes and appreciate all the fresh and glorious days that the summer has to offer.

GENERAL TIPS ON HEALTH AND WELLNESS FOR PITTA TYPE

B elow are some general tips you can adopt in your lifestyle, some of which we've already discussed:

1. The key lifestyle advice to balance Pitta is to stay cool, both physically and emotionally. Avoid going out in the heat of the day, particularly on an empty stomach or after consuming tangy or spicy foods. Avoid workouts when it's hot. Take a walk away from situations that make you heated.
2. Shield yourself from the sun. Keep cool in warm weather by wearing loose cotton clothing. Wear a wide-brimmed cap and shades to shield your eyes while you're out. Drink enough room temperature water.

3. Water-based practices are suitable for Pitta-dominant people. Consider swimming or aqua-aerobics to stay healthy and cool. Strolling after sunset, particularly along the coastline, is also a nice way to bring some leisurely activity into your day.

4. When Pitta is out of balance, you may notice that you fall asleep without much difficulty, but in the very early hours, you wake up and find it hard to get back to sleep. For this, a cup of warm milk with some cardamom can be beneficial before bedtime. It's also crucial to get to bed early, so you can have a good sleep every night.

5. Regular digestion is essential to avoid the build-up of Ama in the body. Triphala Rasayana tends to encourage regularity

and rhythm of the digestive system. Triphala helps improve digestion without aggravating the Pitta Dosha. It also serves to regulate the acid in the stomach.

Because Triphala is gentle, not habit shaping, and not depleting, it can be used repeatedly to maintain regularity.

6. To soothe fragile skin, calm feelings, and nourish and strengthen muscles and nerves, engage in an Ayurvedic massage (Abhyanga) every morning before bathing or showering. Use coconut oil for the massage. If you like, you can add 3-4 drops of pure essential oil like lavender or rose to 2 oz. in Massage oil. Mix before you use it.

Every 2-3 days a week, massage the scalp with warm oil and leave the oil for an hour to two before the shampoo. Apply a pure, soft moisturizer to your body after your shower or bath, or spray your skin with clean rose or sandalwood water to keep your skin feeling cool all day long.

7. Don't skip the food, fast occasionally, and don't wait to eat until you're ravenously hungry. Begin your day with some cooked fruit, accompanied by some cereal. Eat a nourishing meal for lunch and a lighter meal for dinner.

Select sweet juicy fruit for snacking; fully ripe mangoes, sweet pears, and sweet juicy grapes are great Pitta-pacifying options. Delaying meals can induce excess acidity, so you better eat on time every day.

8. Balance work and life. Set aside some time for rest and relaxation every day, don't just get so lost in the job that you can't stay away from it.

9. Set aside approximately 30 minutes per day for meditation, to help balance the heart and feelings, and to improve your body-mind-soul synchronization.

IN A NUTSHELL

A yurvedic texts recommend the concept of opposites to reduce the degree of a dosha that has been exacerbated. As the characteristics of Pitta include lightness, heat, sourness, sharpness, slight unctuousness, and mobility, the attributes that are opposite to these in diet and lifestyle tend to restore equilibrium to Pitta Dosha.

Nourishing Elements: Water, Air, Earth, and Ether

Nourishing Attributes: Cool, Substantial, Aromatic, and Calming

Nourishing Tastes: Sweet, Bitter, and Astringent

Essential Minerals: Copper, Iron, Magnesium, and Potassium

Macronutrients: Carbohydrates 60-70% Protein 20% Fats 10-15%

Functions of Pitta: Sight, Digestion, Temperature, and Appetite.

Locations: Lymphatic System, Blood, Spleen, Liver, Skin, Eyes, and the Heart.

Foods Beneficial to Pitta: Most Beans, Soaked Almonds, and Vegetables.

Food to Avoid: Sour Fruits, Red Meat, Potatoes, Tomatoes, and Eggplant.

Exercise Beneficial to Pitta: A Combination of Rest and a Minimum of 15-20 Minutes of Yoga Every Day are Important to a Pitta Individual.

In each season, the body acts differently. Thus, seasonal practice is essential to maintain well-being and avoid potential seasonal imbalances.

During the transition between hot and cold seasons, the Agni or the digestive fire can start to fluctuate dramatically. If your diet and lifestyle are not compatible with your body type through seasonal changes, the body will be packed with Ama. At the same moment, the Ojas (immune-supporting sap) is reduced. It brings the body in a vulnerable position, increasing the possibilities of illness and diseases.

One of the most important ways to support Pitta is by setting up a routine. The idea of routine goes hand in hand with the physiological clock of the body and the natural cycle of the day. By encouraging routine, we make it possible for our bodies to work in harmony at all times.

Morning Routine

• Begin by getting up at the same time every morning (before 6:00 am to allow the body a chance to be active). Use a small alarm clock if necessary. If you use subtle light prompts and soothing noises, the nervous system is peacefully packed with consciousness. As you wake up, bring your legs to your chest and softly rock back and forth.

• After the feet have hit the floor, drink a glass of warm water with a squeeze of lemon that helps clear the digestive tract and encourages healthy bowel movements.

• Then, perform oil pulling (Keep a tbsp of sesame oil in your mouth and keep swishing it around for at least 10 minutes). During this time you can perform your other morning activities like going to the toilet to ease bodily urges. Lastly, brush your teeth and clean your tongue.

• After that, you should do Abhyanga (Oil Massage) routine, and then take a relaxing bath.

• The morning is the best time to meditate, perform yoga, or exercise. Note that this practice does not need to be a workout if time is not sufficient.

• Take herbs with warm water after this. Then, have your breakfast. Walking after meals improves digestion.

Afternoon

• Remember to eat lunch every day at the same time. Lunch should be enjoyed at noon (12:00 pm to 2:00 pm) and should be the largest meal of the day.

Evening

• Dinner should be served at least 2 hours before bedtime (6:00-8:00 pm), best if consumed before sunset. It ensures that the body is not forced to breakdown food during sleep.

• Gentle stretching before bed will signal to the body that the nervous system is relaxing.

• Take a warm shower or a bath before you lie down to sleep (You can do Abhyanga at night if not during the day). Apply oils to your body and wear comfy clothes that will keep you comfortable throughout the night.

Dietary Recap

Foods that appear to have cool, substantial, aromatic, and calming components reduce Pitta. Below is a recap of the dietary recommendations we discussed.

1. Include a few dry foods in your diet to balance Pitta's liquid nature, some "heavy" foods that provide structure and sustainable nutrition, and foods that are cool to counter Pitta's fiery quality.

2. Choose ghee as your cooking medium in moderate amounts. According to ancient Ayurvedic texts, Ghee cools both the mind and the body. Ghee can be heated to high temperatures without disturbing its nourishing, soothing qualities. So, use ghee to sauté vegetables, spices, or other foods.

3. The 3 Ayurvedic tastes that help control Pitta are sweet, bitter, and astringent, and you can incorporate more of these tastes into your regular diet. Milk, fully ripe sweet fruits, and soaked and blanched almonds make healthy snack options. Eat minimal salty, pungent, and sour tastes.

4. Cooling food is a perfect way to control Pitta Dosha. Sweet juicy fruits, particularly cherries, will cool Pitta quickly. Milk, sweet rice pudding, coconut and coconut juice, and milkshakes produced from ripe mangoes and almonds or dates are examples of Pitta-pacifying foods.

5. Carrots, asparagus, bitter leafy greens, fennel, and cruciferous vegetables—broccoli, cauliflower, brussels sprout, green beans, and bitter gourd—are healthy vegetable options. They are more digestible when are diced and cooked with Pitta-pacifying spices. Vegetables may be mixed with grains or moong beans to accommodate one-course meals.

6. Basmati rice is good for Pitta balancing. Wheat is also good; fresh flatbreads made with whole-wheat flour combine well with cooked vegetables or Pitta-balancing Chutneys (Sauce). Oats and amaranth are two other Pitta-balancing grains.

7. Choose spices that are not too hot or pungent. Ayurvedic spices, such as small quantities of turmeric, cumin, coriander, cinnamon, cardamom, and fennel provide taste, aroma, and soothing wisdom.

8. Drink sweet Lassi in lunch to help improve digestion and cool (not ice-cold) water to quench thirst.

9. Dry cereal, crackers, granola and cereal bars, and rice cakes complement the liquid nature of Pitta Dosha and can be consumed at any time of the day.

By stressing the correct schedule and interacting with the natural cycle of the day, we can promote health. When we adopt a routine schedule, consume nourishing food, and choose to take care of our mind and body, we provide an atmosphere that fosters a calm and balanced Pitta.

YOUR OPINION MATTERS!

Dear Reader,

As you near the conclusion of this book, I'd like to convey my heartfelt appreciation for sticking with me on this journey. I hope the pages you've read have inspired you, taught you insight, and sparked an interest in Ayurvedic lifestyle.

Please consider posting a review on Amazon to share your opinions and experiences. By sharing your review, you not only contribute to common knowledge but also have a significant ripple effect of change and healing in the lives of many readers. Here's a QR that'll take you directly to the review section.

Thank you for your presence, for your support, and for your willingness to start on this transforming journey. May the knowledge contained within these pages continue to resonate deep in your heart and lead you on your road to overall well-being.

Thanks for reading...

You can lend this book to your family, it's free of cost!!

I've made a complete series on these three doshas (Vata, Pitta, and Kapha), one for each. This is Pitta; the other two are also available.

You can also contact me for any queries: rohit@rohitsahu.net or on any of the following social media:

Facebook, Twitter, Instagram, Goodreads, Linkedin

Want to Hear from Me on Ayurveda and Spirituality? - https://rohitsahu.net/join-to-hear/

HERE ARE YOUR
FREE GIFTS!!

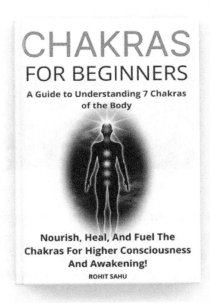

If you're into Chakras and pursuing knowledge about Chakras Awakening and Vibrational Energy, this book will help you pave the way towards your spiritual growth.

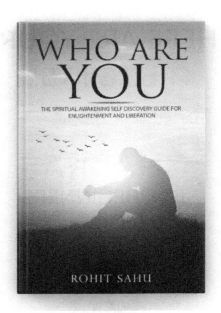

Have you ever thought after reaching your goal, why aren't you happy? It's because that is not what you need to be happy. This is not just another self-help book; this spiritual workbook will help you achieve liberation and be self-enlightened!

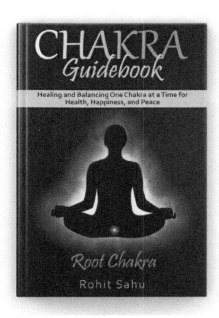

Your 1st Book in the "Chakra Guidebook" series is FREE! This is packed with all the information, tips, and techniques that will make sure that you can effectively heal, balance, and open your Root Chakra.

CLICK HERE to Claim the Books!!

BOOKS BY THIS AUTHOR

Ayurveda For Beginners (3 Book Series)

Ayurveda, which derives from ancient Vedic scriptures, is a 5,000-year-old medical ideology and philosophy based on the idea that we are all made up of different types of energy.

There are three Doshas in Ayurveda that describe the dominant state of mind/body: Vata, Pitta, and Kapha. While all three are present in everyone, Ayurveda suggests that we each have a dominant Dosha that is unwavering from birth, and ideally an equal (though often fluctuating) balance between the other two.

If Doshas are balanced, we are healthy; when they are unbalanced, we develop a disorder commonly expressed by skin problems, impaired nutrition, insomnia, irritability, and anxiety.

Vata, Pitta, and Kapha are all important to our biology in some way, so no one is greater than, or superior to, any other. Each has a very specific set of basic functions to perform in the body.

That said, when the Doshas are out of control, our wellbeing can be damaged. However, before we get into the particulars of each of the three Doshas, it is helpful to understand their basic nature and their wider function in the natural world.

Each of the Doshas has its own special strengths and weaknesses, and with a little awareness, you can do a lot to remain healthy and balanced. You can use this series to adjust your lifestyles and routines in a way that supports your constitution.

I've made a complete series of these three.

Just follow the books along, you'll reveal the easiest step-by-step routine to balance your Dosha by the end of it!

Ayurveda Cookbook For Beginners (3 Book Series)

All you need to know about Ayurvedic diet and cooking along with easy-to-follow recipes backed by the timeless wisdom of Indian heritage to balance your aggravated dosha…

I've made a complete cookbook series on all 3 doshas! You can use this series to adjust your lifestyles and routines in a way that supports your constitution.

With this "Ayurveda Cookbook For Beginners Series," I provide you the best dietary practices, recipes, and everything you need to balance and heal your doshas alongside enjoying the authentic Indian flavors.

This guide's Ayurvedic Cooking techniques tell what to eat and how to eat to help the healing process and assist the body in removing contaminants and maintaining equilibrium. It has a wealth of knowledge on healthy diet, proper food combinations, food quality, food timing, and cooking methods.

All the recipes in this cookbook are traditional, time-tested over decades, and are based on Ayurvedic principles. They can aid a yogi's yoga practice by keeping the mind calm and are thus ideal for all yoga practitioners. The beauty is that the recipes are not only sattvic in nature but are also tasty and have that authentic Indian taste!

Yoga For Beginners (10 Book Series)

Yoga origin can be traced back to more than 5,000 years ago, but some researchers believe that yoga may be up to 10,000 years old. The word 'Yoga' first appeared in the oldest sacred texts, the Rig Veda, and is derived from the Sanskrit root "Yuj" which means to unite.

According to the Yoga Scriptures, the practice of yoga leads an individual to a union of consciousness with that of universal consciousness. It eventually leads to a great harmony between the human mind and body, man, and nature.

Yoga provides multiple health advantages, such as enhancing endurance, reducing depression, and improving overall wellness and fitness.

As yoga has grown into mainstream popularity, many styles and variations have emerged in wellness space. This centuries-old Eastern philosophy is now widely practiced and taught by people of all ages, sizes, and backgrounds.

There are 10 primary types of Yoga. So if you're trying to figure out which of the different types of Yoga is best for you, remember that there's no one right or wrong. You can ask yourself what's important to you in your Yoga practice: Are you searching for a sweaty, intense practice, or are you searching for a more meditative, gentler practice that looks more appealing?

Like you choose any sort of exercise, choose something you want to do.

Here's a complete series on all 10 types of yoga.

This guide can be used by beginners, advanced students, teachers, trainees, and teacher training programs. Covering the fundamentals of each pose in exact detail, including how to correct the most common mistakes, as well as changes to almost all body types, this yoga guides has left nothing to help you make daily breakthroughs.

Ayurvedic Weight Loss Guide: Lose Weight The Healthy Way As Per Ayurveda

Are you sick of pursuing diet after diet without ever reaching your target weight? Perhaps you're just ready for a more holistic approach to weight loss, or you're trying to reset after feeling out of sync with your diet or lifestyle for a short period of time.

Ayurveda offers a straightforward, achievable, and practical approach to weight loss. You'll also be regaining a vibrant feeling of health and well-being along the way. It is always unfailing, consistent, and dependable, as well as incredibly simple to implement.

Ayurvedic weight loss methods may naturally lead us towards holistic and healthy living with no artificial or processed foods or fad diets that damage us more than they help.

A considerable quantity of evidence supports these practices and their significance for weight loss and healthy living. Living an Ayurvedic lifestyle will improve your health and make you more conscious of what you eat, how you move, and how you feel.

This Ayurvedic Weight Loss Guide Covers:
✓Introduction to Ayurveda
✓Reasons for Losing Weight Other than Cosmetic Purposes
✓Common Issues with Diets
✓Ayurveda on Weight Loss
✓Key to Ayurveda's Weight Loss Success
✓Ayurvedic Weight Loss Practices
✓The Role of Routine for Weight Loss

✓Herbs to Boost Your Progress
✓Common Myths and FAQs

So, if you're willing to give an entirely different approach a go, be ready to embark on a new connection with your body as well as an impactful path toward better overall health.

Welcome to the Ayurvedic weight loss approach. This is something you can do. In fact, it may enrich your life in ways that no previous "diet" has ever done.

Slowly but surely, Ayurvedic knowledge will guide you toward stress-free, healthy weight loss.

Reiki For Beginners: The Step-By-Step Guide To Unlock Reiki Self-Healing And Aura Cleansing Secrets For Deep Healing, Peace Of Mind, And Spiritual Growth

Have you always been curious about Reiki? Do you want to witness Reiki in action? Or have you already started your Reiki practice but are looking for additional info? If that's the case, this book is jam-packed with the knowledge that will offer you all you need to know about Reiki so that you may enjoy the benefits of this wonderful practice in your life.

With all the business and technology in our life these days, it is quite simple to have blocked energy. We may be upset about something, neglect our relationships, and do numerous other things. All of this may lead to a variety of physical illnesses and other issues that will not allow us to live healthy or happy life. We may open up our energy and enable it to flow freely through the body using Reiki.

This beginner's guide aims to educate you on how to soothe your mind, body, and soul. You'll be able to ignite your energy and find a strong route to self-attunement and beyond! You will also develop great intuition and clarity, bringing you closer to your inner and spiritual vigor.

This handbook discusses Reiki and how beneficial it may be. Reiki is all around us, and everyone may benefit from its warm, loving energy to help with balance and healing. Because the corpus of information on this topic is so vast, I attempted to condense hundreds of lessons and readings into one easy-to-read book. This book will get you started with Reiki, from the Reiki Symbolism and hand postures through a comprehensive explanation of the various Reiki Techniques.

It will go into how Reiki is an excellent method for moving and healing the energy within our chakras. Reiki practice may cure and reduce pain, both mental and physical, by utilizing vibrations and warmth. You will also have the skills to alter the lives of others if you learn it, and there is nothing more beautiful than compassionate love and healing.

Consider this book to be your insightful Reiki teacher, leading you along your Reiki path to nurture healing. This complete guide includes simple and inclusive training that is comprehensible and accessible to everyone, as well as instructive pictures and guidance that make this book ideal for Reiki students of any age or background.

With this book, you can learn:
✓What Exactly is Reiki?
✓Basics, History, and Principles of Reiki
✓The Energy Centers (Chakras), Their Functioning, and Imbalances
✓The Fundamentals and Knowhow of Kundalini
✓The Meridians in Your Body, How They Interconnect and Affect Us

✓Methods for Resolving Symptoms of Obstructed Energy in Your Mind and Body
✓Reiki's Foundational Pillars
✓The Reiki Advantages
✓Reiki Hand Postures
✓Step-by-Step Reiki Healing
✓Healing Others
✓Reiki Symbols that have the Powerful Healing Forces with Them
✓How Reiki May Significantly Improve Your Health
✓Aura Cleanse and How to Perform An Aura Scan to Feel the Energy in Your Body
✓The Amazing Properties of Crystals and How They Can Boost Your Reiki Practice
✓Tips to Boost Your Reiki Growth
✓Reiki's Most Common FAQs and Myths

Thus, if you are ready to cleanse your energy and experience the happiness and good health that you have been seeking without the use of physicians and medicine, be sure to read this book and learn all you need to get started with Reiki! Don't worry if you're not sure where to begin with spiritual healing. This book will guide you through the recovery process step by step, at your own pace!

More significantly, you will learn how to cleanse your aura and release negativity to promote the universal life force inside your body.

Vipassana Meditation: The Buddhist Mindfulness Practice To Cultivate Joy, Peace, Calmness, And Awakening!!

Are you looking to cultivate true unconditional love towards the creation and experience utter bliss? Do you wish to foster resilience, non-judgment, and detachment? Will you like to master the ancient mindfulness technique that leaded Gautama Buddha to Enlightenment/Nirvana? Do you want to promote relaxation, mindfulness, gratitude, and a better sense of inner peace? Do you want to witness the joy of living in the present moment? If so, Vipassana Meditation is what you need...

Vipassana, which means "seeing things as they really are," is an Indian and Buddhist meditation practice. It was taught over 2500 years ago as a generic cure for universal maladies, i.e., an Art of Living. It is a simple knowledge of what is happening as it is happening.

It is distinct from other forms of meditation practices. The bulk of meditations, whether on a mantra, flame, or activity such as Trataka, are focused on concentration. The practitioner directs his mental energy on an item or a concept. Such methods have validity in terms of relaxing the mind, relaxation, a feeling of well-being, stress reduction, and so on.

Vipassana, in contrast to the other practices, focuses on awareness rather than concentration. Vipassana refers to perceiving reality as it is rather than changing reality, as in concentration practices. The key attribute of Vipassana is its secular nature, which allows it to be practiced by people of any religion, race, caste, nationality, or gender. If the method is to be universal, it must be used by everyone. Here, you concentrate on your breathing, and as you gain control of your breathing observation, you move on to your body responses.

The more the method is used, the more freedom from suffering there is, and the closer one gets to the ultimate objective of complete liberation. Even 10 days may provide effects that are apparent and clearly helpful in daily life.

This step-by-step Vipassana guide takes the reader through

practices that may open new levels of awareness and understanding. This book's aim is to teach you how to live consciously so that you may ultimately be calm and joyful every day of your life!

This is an authentic and practical guide to samatha, materialism, mind, dependent origination, and Vipassana based on the Buddha's teachings. This book will walk you through the stages and methods of overcoming stress, sadness, fear, and anxiety through the practice of Vipassana meditation.

It will explain what this method is and how it came to be. This book also demonstrates how to utilize Vipassana meditation to make our everyday lives more meaningful and, ultimately, to discover the real meaning of peace and tranquillity.

In this book, you'll discover:
✓History of Vipassana Meditation
✓The Deeper Realm of Vipassana
✓The Purpose of Vipassana
✓The Benefits of Vipassana Meditation
✓The Right Attitude Towards the Practice
✓How to Create a Vipassana Retreat at Home
✓The Step-By-Step Vipassana Meditation Practice
✓Tips to Boost Your Progress
✓Additions to Catalyze Your Vipassana Session
✓Beginners Mistakes
✓Common Myths and FAQs
✓Some Pointers from My Experience

Following the instructions in this book will teach you how to develop profound stability, maintain an in-depth study of the intricacies of mind and matter, and ultimately unravel deeply conditioned patterns that perpetuate suffering. It acknowledges with a detailed examination of the different insight and spiritual fruits that the practice offers, Nirvana/Enlightenment being the end goal.

Aromatherapy To Foster Health, Beauty, Healing, And Well-Being!!

Do you want to fill your home with calming essence and the pleasant smell of nature? Do you wish to get rid of stress and anxiety and relieve various physical and mental conditions? Are you looking to improve your overall physical, mental, emotional, and spiritual health? Do you wish to escalate your spiritual practices? If so, Aromatherapy is what you need...

Even though the word "Aromatherapy" was not coined until the late 1920s, this kind of therapy was found many centuries earlier. The history of the use of essential oils traces back to at least a few thousand years, although human beings have used plants, herbs, etc. for thousands of years. They have been used to improve a person's health or mood for over 6,000 years. Its roots may be traced back to ancient Egypt when fragrant compounds like frankincense and myrrh were utilized in religious and spiritual rituals.

Aromatherapy, often known as essential oil treatment, refers to a group of traditional, alternative, and complementary therapies that make use of essential oils and other aromatic plant components. It is a holistic therapeutic therapy that promotes health and well-being by using natural plant extracts. It employs the therapeutic use of fragrant essential oils to enhance the health of the body, mind, and soul.

Various techniques are used to extract essential or volatile oils from the plant's flowers, bark, stems, leaves, roots, fruits, and other components. It arose as a result of scientists deciphering the antibacterial and skin permeability characteristics of essential oils.

In the modern world, aromatherapy and essential oils have become increasingly popular, not only in the usage of aromatherapy massage and the purchase of pure essential oils but also in the extensive use of essential oils in the cosmetic, skincare, and pharmaceutical industries. Aromatherapy is considered both an art and a science. It provides a variety of medical and psychological advantages, depending on the essential oil or oil combination and manner of application employed.

With this book, I'll share with you every aspect of aromatherapy, as well as the finest techniques you may use to reap the physical, mental, emotional, and spiritual benefits.

This book brings light to the world of aromatherapy by offering a wealth of knowledge and practical guidance on how to get the most out of essential oils. It will offer the best option for living a joyful, natural, healthy, and homeopathic way of life. You will discover a variety of information on the best aromatherapy oils on these pages, including benefits, tips, applications, precautions, myths, and FAQs for using them safely and effectively.

You will discover the science of aromatherapy and how essential oils may totally change your well-being by using the methods mentioned. This book will help you use these potent plant extracts to start feeling better inside and out, no matter where you are on your aromatherapy self-care journey.

In this book, you'll discover:
✓What is Aromatherapy?
✓History and its Significance
✓Aromatherapy Benefits and Conditions it may Treat
✓What are Essential Oils?
✓How are Essential oils Made?

✓The Best Storage Procedure
✓How to Buy Quality Essential Oils?
✓The Best Way to Perform Aromatherapy
✓Activities to perform with Aromatherapy
✓Some Tips that'll Boost Your Progress
✓Essential Oils to Avoid
✓Safety and Precautions
✓Myths and FAQs

So, if you are interested in healing with minimum medication use, spending your time learning about essential oils is a good place to start. Just stick with me until the end to discover how this becomes your ultimate aromatherapy reference and the manifestation of your motives.

The Ayurvedic Dinacharya: Master Your Daily Routine As Per Ayurveda For A Healthy Life And Well-Being!!

Do you wish to synchronize your schedule with nature's rhythm? Do you wish to be disease-free for the rest of your life? Do you want to live a longer, better, and happier life? If yes, this book is going to be an important asset in your life...

Our generation is usually always going through a tough phase. Late nights at work, early meetings, and hectic social life are just a few things that add to our everyday stress. But the main cause for your distress is the lack of a regular schedule. Our forefathers never had to worry about stress since they maintained a disciplined Dinacharya that they followed faithfully. This helps keep the doshas in balance, controls the body's biological cycle, promotes discipline and happiness, and reduces stress.

A lack of routine can also cause many lifestyle disorders such as obesity, hypertension and stroke, diabetes, coronary heart disease, dyslipidemia, cancer, arthritis, anxiety, insomnia, constipation, indigestion, hyperacidity, gastric ulcer, and early manifestations of aging like greying of hair, wrinkles, depletion of energy levels, etc. Simple adjustments in one's lifestyle may prevent these numerous health risks and more.

Dinacharya is formed from two words—'Dina,' which means day, and 'Acharya,' which means activity. By incorporating Dinacharya's basic self-care practices into your life, you will be armed with the skills you need to foster balance, joy, and overall long-term health. It teaches people how to live a better, happier, and longer life while avoiding any illnesses. So irrespective of your body type, age, gender, or health condition, you should opt for a healthy lifestyle.

A daily routine is essential for bringing about a dramatic transformation in the body, mind, and consciousness. Routine aids in the establishment of equilibrium in one's constitution. It also helps with digestion, absorption, and assimilation, as well as generating self-esteem, discipline, tranquility, happiness, and longevity.

With this book, I'll show you how to align yourself with nature's rhythm every day so you may remain healthy and happy for the rest of your life. You will overcome all kinds of mental and physical illnesses in your life. The best part is that these suggestions are centered on Ayurvedic principles and are easy to implement.

This book covers:
✓What is Dinacharya?
✓Importance of Dinacharya
✓Dinacharya Benefits
✓Daily Cycles and Dinacharya
✓The Morning Dinacharya
✓The Afternoon and Sundown Dinacharya

✓The Evening and Night Dinacharya
✓How to Implement Dinacharya into Your Life?
✓Tips to Boost Your Progress
✓Beginners Dinacharya Mistakes

This book is perfect for anybody seeking simple, all-encompassing methods to live a more genuine and balanced life. You'll discover techniques and ideas to help you stay calm, balanced, and joyful.

Shadow Work For Beginners: A Short And Powerful Guide To Make Peace With Your Hidden Dark Side That Drive You And Illuminate The Hidden Power Of Your True Self For Freedom And Lasting Happiness

Do you want to recognize and heal the shadow patterns and wounds of your inner child? Do you wish to get rooted in your soul for wholeness? Do you want to influence your programs and beliefs to attain eternal bliss? Do you want to know where you are on the ladder of consciousness, and how to move up? Do you want to learn how to forgive, let go, and have compassion for yourself and others? Do you want to alter and strengthen your mindset to maximize every aspect of your life? If so, this guide is just what you need.

For many, the word "shadow work" conjures up all sorts of negative and dark ideas. Because of the beliefs we have of the term shadow, it is tempting to believe that shadow work is a morbid spiritual practice or that it is an internal work that includes the more destructive or evil facets of our personalities. But that's not the case. In fact, shadow work is vital to your spiritual growth. When you go through a spiritual awakening, there comes a point where "shadow work" becomes necessary. So, what exactly is the 'Human Shadow,' and what is 'Shadow

Work?'

The definition of the shadow self is based on the idea that we figuratively bury certain bits of personality that we feel will not be embraced, approved, or cherished by others; thus, we hold them in the "shadows." In brief, our shadows are the versions of ourselves that we do not offer society.

It includes aspects of our personality that we find shameful, unacceptable, ugly. It may be anger, resentment, frustration, greed, hunger for strength, or the wounds of childhood—all those we hold secret. You might claim it's the dark side of yourself. And no matter what everyone suggests, they all have a dark side of their personalities.

Shadow Work is the practice of loving what is, and of freeing shame and judgment, so that we can be our true self in order to touch the very depths of our being, that is what Shadow Work means. You have to dwell on the actual problems rather than on past emotions. If you do so, you get to the problems that have you stressed out instantly and easily. And to be at peace, we need to get in touch with our darker side, rather than suppressing it.

Whether you have struggled with wealth, weight, love, or something else, after dissolving the shadows within, you will find that your life is transforming in both tiny and drastic ways. You'll draw more optimistic people and better opportunities. Your life will be nicer, easier, and even more abundant.

The book covers the easiest practices and guided meditation to tap into the unconscious. It's going to help you explore certain aspects so that they will no longer control your emotions. Just imagine what it would be if you could see challenges as exciting obstacles rather than experiencing crippling anxiety.

This book is going to be the Momentum you need to get to where you're trying to be. You'll go deeper into your thoughts, the beliefs that hold you back disappear, and you get a head start on your healing journey.

In this guide, you'll discover:

✓What is the Human Shadow?
✓Characteristics of Shadow
✓Do We All Have a Shadow Self?
✓How is The Shadow Born?
✓What is the Golden Shadow?
✓The Mistake We All Make
✓What is Shadow Work?
✓Benefits of Shadow Work
✓Tips on Practicing Shadow Work
✓Shadow Work Stages
✓Shadow Work Techniques and Practices
✓Shadow Work Mindfulness
✓Shadow Work FAQs

Covering every bit of Shadow Work, this guide will subtly reveal the root of your fear, discomfort, and suffering, showing you that when you allow certain pieces of yourself to awaken and be, you will eventually begin to recover, transcend your limits, and open yourself to the light and beauty of your true existence.

Spiritual Empath: The Ultimate Guide To Awake Your Maximum Capacity And Have That Power, Compassion, And Wisdom Contained In Your Soul

Do you keep attracting toxic individuals and set a poor barrier? Do you get consumed by negative emotions and feel like you can't deal with it? Do you want to heal yourself and seek inner peace and spiritual growth? If so, this book is going to open the doors for you!!

Empaths have too much to contribute as healers, creators, friends, lovers, and innovators at work. Yet extremely compassionate and empathic people sometimes give too much at the cost of their own well-being-and end up consuming the stress of others. Why?

These questions and more will be addressed in this book. You'll find the answers you're searching for to learn the facts on whether you're an empath, how it can work on a biological level, what to do to help you succeed as an empath, and how to shield yourself from other people's thoughts, feelings, and responses so that you don't absorb them.

There is a lot of things going in the life of empaths, and they are here to add more happiness and peace to the world. Empaths are known for their willingness to listen, sensitivity, empathy, and the capacity to be in the shoes of others. You may be that individual, or you might know that individual in your life, but either way, knowing the true cause of being an empath and why they are different from others will help you improve to lead a healthy, free, and beautiful life full of empathy.

This book includes the following, and much more:

✓What is an Empath?
✓Are You an Empath?
✓Is Being an Empath a Gift or Disorder
✓The List of Empath Superpowers
✓Ways to Turn Your Super Traits into Super Powers
✓The Secret Dark Side of Being an Empath
✓What It's Like Being an Intuitive/Psychic Empath
✓Signs You're the Most Powerful Empath (Heyoka)
✓Is Your Soul Exhausted and Energy Depleted?
✓Tips To Become an Empath Warrior
✓Empath's Survival Guide/Tips to Stay Balanced as an Empath

✓Ways to Save Yourself from Narcissists
✓Best Practices to Deal with Anxiety
✓Why Self-Love/Self-Care is So Important
✓Empath Awakening Stages
✓Best Transmutation Techniques for Raising Your Energies and Vibrations for Spiritual Growth

Right now, you can opt to proceed on a profound healing path and find strength in the deep pockets of your soul. Or you might want to put off the re-discovery of your inner voice and intuition, feeling like you might never have had it; never really understood how your powerful empathic ability can be channeled for the greatest benefit of all, including your own highest gain.

Filled with lots of insight into the inner workings of Empath's mind, useful knowledge to help you make sense of your abilities, and keep negative individuals and energies out of your life. This book contains all you need to become a stronger, better version of yourself.

That's correct, with this book, you can move out of your usual role and begin a journey. You'll experience the emergence of the inner energies and become a spiritually awakened person.

Meditation For Beginners: The Easiest Guide To Cultivate Awareness, Acceptance, And Peace To Unleash Your Inner Strength And Explore The Deepest Realm Of Your Being!!

Whether you're looking to increase self-awareness, reduce negative emotions, bust stress, promote creativity, foster good health and mental peace, or transcend the limitations of human life and connect with universal forces to see the transcendental reality through it (called Brahman in the Vedas), meditation solves all...

It is estimated that 200–500 million individuals meditate across the globe. Meditation statistics suggest that the practice has grown in popularity in recent years. Given all the health advantages it provides, it's no wonder that a rising number of individuals are using it. Through it, more and more people are recognizing a profound inner longing for authenticity, connection, compassion, and aliveness.

Meditation may seem to be a simple concept—sit still, focus on your breath, and observe. However, the practice of meditation has a long cultural history that has seen it evolve from a religious concept to something that might today seem more alluring than spiritual. It is a centuries-old technique that is said to have started in India thousands of years ago. Throughout history, the practice was gradually adopted by neighboring nations and became a part of numerous religions around the globe.

The goal of meditation is to become consciously aware of or explore one's own mind and body to get to know oneself. It is fundamentally both an exclusive and inclusive process in which one withdraws one's thoughts and senses from the distractions of the world and concentrates on a selected object or idea.

It is focused attention, with or without an individual's will, in which the mind and body must be brought together to work as one harmonic whole. We may overcome mental obstacles, negative thinking, crippling worries, tension, and anxiety with the aid of meditation by understanding and dealing with the underlying causes. We gain insightful awareness in meditation, allowing us to manage our responses and reactions.

So, whether you want to ease stress, attain spiritual enlightenment, seek peace, or flow through movement, meditation is the way to go.

But how will we know which meditation practice is best for us as there are plenty of them?? While there are various types of meditation, each takes you to the same spot. It's like there are various routes to the same destination. So, it didn't matter which route you take. Here in this book, I'll discuss a certain type of meditation that I found to be the easiest and most effective.

Although there is no right or incorrect method to meditate, it is important to select a practice that matches your requirements and compliments your nature. And the type of meditation I'm going to discuss here is ideal for anyone—from beginners to advanced.

The practice will inject far-reaching and long-lasting advantages into your life—lower stress, more awareness of your struggles, better ability to connect, enhanced awareness, and being nicer to yourself are just some of its benefits.

In this book, you'll discover:
✓What is Meditation?
✓Meditation Benefits
✓The Role of Diet in Meditation
✓Various Mudras
✓Various Asanas
✓The Ideal Setting for Meditation
✓How Yoga and Pranayamas can Help Boost the Practice?
✓The Easiest Meditation Practice
✓The Wrong Way to Approach Meditation
✓The Right Way to Approach Meditation
✓The Significance of Keeping the Spine Straight
✓The Importance of Breath Rhythm
✓Some Tips to Enhance the Practice
✓How Group Meditation is Better than Meditating Alone?
✓The Significance of Routine

✓How to Bring Meditation to Daily Life Activities?
✓Common Meditation Myths and FAQs
✓Some Tips from Experience

So, if you're ready, claim your copy right now and embark on this quest beyond yourself...

Who Are You: The Spiritual Awakening Self Discovery Guide For Enlightenment And Liberation (Available For Free!!)

Have you ever thought after reaching your goal, why aren't you happy? It's because that is not what you need to be happy.

The major problem today in this world is that everyone is searching for joy in materialistic objects like money, fame, respect, and whatever. But the fact is, the most successful personalities in the world which you admire so much are not happy at all! If that was the case, they won't ever get depressed or sad. Is that what the reality is? No, in fact, they're the one who takes depression therapies and drugs to be happy.

What are all the fundamental problems that we all face? There is a sense of lack that exists in all of us, a sense of loneliness, a sense of incompleteness, a sense of being restricted, a sense of fear, fear of death. So these fundamental problems can only be overcome through self-investigation; there's no other way around.

Being happy is a basic nature of human beings, just like the basic nature of fire is hot. But the error we make is we're searching for happiness outside, which is impossible to achieve. Say, you wanted something for a very long time; what happens after you achieve it? You'll be happy for a while, but then you'll need something else to be happy, you'll then run after some other goal; it's an endless cycle!

The good thing is, there's a way to be happy at every moment, but to make it happen you must understand in a peaceful state of mind "Who Are You?"
You'll have to self-enquire! This book is based on one of the most popular Indian Scripture "Ashtavakra Geeta" that reveals the ultimate truth of mankind. It will open the doors for you on how we can achieve self-knowledge and be fearless. All your fears and doubts will come to an end; not temporarily, but forever. All internal conflicts will fall to zero, and psychological pain will cease to exist.

This is not just another self-help book; this spiritual workbook will help you achieve liberation and be self-enlightened!

Reading this book:
✓You'll attain everlasting peace
✓You'll understand the real meaning of spiritual awakening
✓You'll understand spirituality over religion
✓You'll get the answer to 'Who Are You?'
✓You'll be fearless
✓You'll be free from bondage and be able to achieve liberation
✓You'll get the key to everlasting happiness and joy
✓You'll grasp the real essence of spirituality and the awakening self
✓You'll get to know about spirituality for the skeptic
✓You'll discover your higher self
✓You'll be able to experience the joy of self-realization
✓You'll find what spiritual enlightenment means in Buddhism
✓You'll know how to achieve or reach spiritual enlightenment
✓You'll know what happens after spiritual enlightenment
✓You'll get the answer to why you should have spiritual awakening

And this is a book not just for adults but also for kids and teens.

Chakras For Beginners: A Guide To Understanding 7 Chakras Of The Body: Nourish, Heal, And Fuel The Chakras For Higher Consciousness And Awakening! (Available For Free!!)

Chakras are the circular vortexes of energy that are placed in seven different points on the spinal column, and all the seven chakras are connected to the various organs and glands within the body. These chakras are responsible for disturbing the life energy, which is also known as Qi or Praana.

Chakras have more than one dimension to them. One dimension is their physical existence, but they also have a spiritual dimension. Whenever a chakra is disrupted or blocked, the life energy also gets blocked, leading to the onset of mental and health ailments. When the harmonious balance of the seven chakras is disrupted or damaged, it can cause several problems in our lives, including our physical health, emotional health, and our mental state of mind. If all our chakras are balanced and in harmony, our body will function in an optimum way; If unbalanced, our energies will be like in a small river where the water will flow irregularly and noisily. By balancing our chakras, the water/our energies will flow more freely throughout our bodies and thus the risk of imbalances and consequent illnesses will be reduced to a minimum.

In this book, I'm going to give you an excellent resource you can use to amplify the work you do with your chakras.

In this book you'll learn:

✓The Number of Chakras in Our Body (Not 7)
✓The Location of Chakras

✓Meaning Related to Each Chakra
✓Color Psychology
✓How to Balance the Chakras
✓Characteristics/Impacts of Each Chakra When Balanced and Imbalanced
✓Aspects of Nature
✓Qualities
✓Gemstones to Support Each Chakra

Step-By-Step Beginners Instant Pot Cookbook (Vegan): 100+ Easy, Delicious Yet Extremely Healthy Instant Pot Recipes Backed By Ayurveda Which Anyone Can Make In Less Than 30 Minutes

Who said healthy foods can't be tasty, I am a health-conscious person and love to eat healthy food, as well as tasty food.

"You Don't Have to Cook Fancy or Complicated Masterpieces. Just Tasty Food From Simple Healthy Ingredients."

Well, you don't have to struggle anymore with the taste. Here in this cookbook, you'll find 100+ easy yet extremely delicious instant pot recipes. keeping in mind the health factor, all these recipes are backed by Ayurveda, so yes, all are highly nutritious as well.

If you follow Ayurveda you know why we shouldn't eat meat or non-veg, so finally here is a Complete Vegan Instant Pot Cookbook. Plus, these do not require ingredients that'll hurt your budget, nearly all the ingredients are readily available in your home.

Every recipe is properly portioned and will be ready in 30 minutes or less. These quick and simple recipes will get your meal ready on the table in no time.

In this Instant Pot Cookbook you will find:

✓ Insider's Knowledge on How to Make the Most Out of Your Instant Pot
✓ Common FAQs and Other Must-Know Facts about Your Instant Pot
✓ Pro Tips to Get the Most out of Your Instant pot
✓ Things Not to Do with Your Instant Pot
✓ No Non-Veg, Complete Vegan Recipes
✓ How to Create a Variety of Healthy, Easy-to-Make, Delicious Recipes in the Easiest Way Possible

No matter if you're a solo eater, or if you cook for the whole family or friends, with these easy and healthy recipes, you can surprise your family, friends, and your loved ones.

This cookbook includes delicious recipes for:

✓Breakfast Meals
✓Stews and Chilies
✓Soups
✓Beans
✓Lunch/Brunch
✓Side Meals
✓Main Course Meals
✓Appetizers & Snacks
✓Light Dinner
✓Deserts
✓Bonus Recipes Including Salads, Drinks, and Some of the Most Popular Indian Dishes